Natural Methods for Equine Health

Other horse books from Blackwell Science

The Equine Athlete
How to Develop your Horse's
Athletic Potential
Jo Hodges and Sarah Pilliner
0 632 03506 4

Getting Horses Fit
A Guide to
Improving Performance
Second Edition
Sarah Pilliner
0 632 03476 9

Horse and Stable Management
Second Edition
Jeremy Houghton Brown and
Vincent Powell-Smith
0 632 03594 3

Horse Care
Jeremy Houghton Brown and
Sarah Pilliner
0 632 03551 X

Equine Injury, Therapy and
Rehabilitation
Second Edition
Mary Bromiley
0 632 03608 7

Keeping Horses
The Working Owner's Guide to
Saving Time and Money
Second Edition
Susan McBane
0 632 03443 2

Coaching the Rider
Jane Houghton Brown
0 632 03931 0

Breeding the Competition Horse
Second Edition
John Rose and Sarah Pilliner
0 632 03727 X

The Competition Horse
Breeding, Production and
Management
Susan McBane and Gillian McCarthy
0 632 02327 9

Horse Business Management
Second Edition
Jeremy Houghton Brown and
Vincent Powell-Smith
0 632 03821 7

Veterinary Manual for the
Performance Horse
N. S. Loving and A. M. Johnston
0 632 03914 0

Natural Methods for Equine Health

Mary W. Bromiley
FCSP, SRP, RPT (USA)
Chartered Physiotherapist

Illustrations by Camille and Penelope Slattery

Photography by S. Bartlegg

Blackwell Science

© Mary Bromiley 1994

Blackwell Science Ltd
Editorial Offices:
Osney Mead, Oxford OX2 0EL
25 John Street, London WC1N 2BL
23 Ainslie Place, Edinburgh EH3 6AJ
238 Main Street, Cambridge
    Massachusetts 02142, USA
54 University Street, Carlton
    Victoria 3053, Australia

Other Editorial Offices:
Arnette Blackwell SA
  1, rue de Lille
  75007 Paris
  France

Blackwell Wissenschafts-Verlag GmbH
  Kurfürstendamm 57
  10707 Berlin
  Germany

  Feldgasse 13
  A-1238 Wien
  Austria

First published 1994
Reprinted 1995, 1996

Set by DP Photosetting, Aylesbury, Bucks
Printed and bound in Great Britain by
Hartnolls Limited, Bodmin, Cornwall

DISTRIBUTORS
Marston Book Services Ltd
PO Box 87
Oxford OX2 0DT
(*Orders:* Tel: 01865 791155
          Fax: 01865 791927
          Telex: 837515)

USA
Blackwell Science, Inc.
238 Main Street,
Cambridge, MA 02142
(*Orders:* Tel: 800 215-1000
              617 876-7000
          Fax: 617 492-5263)

Canada
Oxford University Press
70 Wynford Drive
Don Mills
Ontario M3C 1J9
(*Orders:* Tel: 416 441-2941)

Australia
Blackwell Science Pty Ltd
54 University Street
Carlton, Victoria 3053
(*Orders:* Tel: 03 347-0300
          Fax: 03 349-3016)

A catalogue record for this book is available
from the British Library

ISBN 0–632–03818–7

Library of Congress
Cataloging in Publication Data
is available

---

*Dedicated to the memory of my mother and her mother both of
whom presented the search of knowledge as exciting*

Contents

Preface

As the end of the twentieth century approaches it seems incredible that at its beginning a 'horseless' way of life was, to the majority of the populace unthinkable. Every man, woman and child, no matter what their station within the community, was in daily contact with horses. For those who worked with or owned a horse its health and well being were of paramount importance, and 'horse lore' had been handed down from generation to generation.

Chemical medicine, as we use it today, was unthought of. The remedies to combat problems were concocted from substances supplied from natural resources: mustard, camphor, ginger, peppermint oil, linseed, mercury, arsenic, to name but a few. Feed additives were also natural – a sod of turf, a mangel (a root vegetable rarely grown today), a pinch of nitre, furze (gorse), and so on.

In 1894 George Armitage, MRCVS, devoted a section of his book, *The Horse, Management in Health and Disease*, to The Stable. He discussed aspect, drainage, ventilation, paving, and stable utensils. In a further section he gave detailed descriptions of feeding horses both stabled and at pasture, watering and grooming. Interestingly, he said the latter should be done 'first thing in the morning' and then the box 'set fair'. Few modern books on husbandry take such a detailed approach.

The horse population declined as engines took over, and two world wars radically changed the lifestyle of the majority of the populace. Since the end of World War II the horse has regained its place in the community. Numbers have increased to make equine recreation and its associated trades the largest of the leisure industries. Many people with no traditional knowledge now own horses. All wish to keep their horses healthy and happy. Most available literature tends to describe what to do after something has gone wrong, but this book seeks to discuss those methods which aim to keep all the components from which the horse is constructed in balance or harmony – methods which have stood the test of time. It is important to adopt the philosophy of regarding 'the whole', not the particular, for any problem will always create secondary effects.

One factor which must be accepted is that changes have taken place during the twentieth century which could never have been envisaged at its beginning, let alone by the Egyptians who were the first at around 8000 BC to document disease, suggest remedies, and advocate massage for health. We have no idea if the dreaded viral invasions were present as long ago as 8000 BC, and despite all our modern knowledge we as yet have no methods to enable us to influence the defence systems of the body to combat such invasions. This is still a challenge which awaits answers!

It should be appreciated that the therapies we describe today as 'complementary' or 'alternative' (to chemicals) were originally developed to deal with the problems experienced in an earlier time which was vastly different to the chemically polluted environment in which we now try to exist. The current environmental conditions could explain the apparent lack of success experienced by some who go 'alternative'.

Chinese physicians were only paid if their patrons remained in good health. As a modern follow-up to this attitude, this book will, in the main, discuss ways of promoting good health, rather than listing ways to cure poor health.

The first part of the book discusses the general structure and organization of the body, as well as the nutritional benefits of herbs, vitamins and minerals. The second part, *Therapies*, gives information about homoeopathy, acupuncture and acupressure, and how these can be related to your horse. The concluding section is devoted to massage and stretches. I have included here detailed information on muscles and their potential problems, as well as general points and exercises for those who wish to undertake horse massage.

Acknowledgements

My grateful thanks are due to many people too numerous to mention by name who have criticized, encouraged, and freely exchanged experience and knowledge. However I would like to specially single out a few: the late Stella Parker of the Turks and Caicos Islands for her insight into herbs; the late Marjorie Blackie for introducing me to homoeopathy; and Saied Longe, one time senior staff nurse at Sungei

Buloh Leper Colony in Malaya, who exposed me to traditional Chinese acupuncture. Thanks are also due to my secretary Sue Langfrey who has uncomplainingly deciphered my writing and created order out of chaos.

Mary W. Bromiley

Part I
The Body and Nutrition

1 Organization of the Body

Introduction

The key to success in any situation is understanding. A basic knowledge of the structure of the horse will help you to appreciate the complexity of the interaction between the various systems of the body and the ingredients which need to be assembled and assimilated to maintain the living being. It is also important to have an awareness of the problems that can occur should the normal interaction between cells or body systems cease or become ineffective.

Before we discuss the individual components and body systems try to visualize the whole. Think first of a motor car: it is assembled and leaves the production line as a usable object provided it has air in its tyres, the correct oil and fuel in the appropriate systems, and water. Malfunctions occur if any of these needs are not met – a diesel engine performs poorly if fed petrol, the engine performs poorly if not fed oil, overheating occurs if the water does not circulate and cool the system, and so on. From time to time parts wear out and need to be replaced. Switch to the horse – a living object complete at birth but not yet grown to full size. The car and the horse differ: the car is constructed in a factory while the horse is developed by the workings of its own internal 'factories', *but* both require raw materials to be present in the correct quantities for the factories to be able to manufacture their units.

Cells

Cells are the basic unit of all life. They are controlled by, and will respond to, electrical, chemical and magnetic stimuli. Life begins with the meeting of a sperm and an ova, and the resulting single fertilized cell divides and sub-divides forming a fetus. The raw materials required for this process are absorbed from the blood of the mare which, during pregnancy, passes through the placenta. Unwanted substances cannot pass through the walls of the placental vessels and are effectively filtered out lest they harm the growing fetus. It is obvious that if the mare is able to find, or is fed, the required ingredients for the growing fetus, the foal, when finally born, will be healthy and the mare's milk will contain the nutrients needed by the foal. A mare who fares badly during pregnancy will be forced to draw upon her own internal reserves, thus she becomes weak and may deliver an undernourished foal. Therefore problems may have their beginnings *in utero*.

While this brief discussion of fetal development may seem to have moved away from cell structure, an appreciation of the fact 'that what you do not put in will not come out' is very important to the text.

As the original cell divides and sub-divides into literally millions of new cells, differentiation takes place and cells remodel to exhibit characteristics peculiar to their eventual function as a body tissue or system. Cells have a number of fascinating aspects:

● Each individual cell is as complex as a galaxy in space.
● Each type of body tissue exhibits a particular cell clumping or

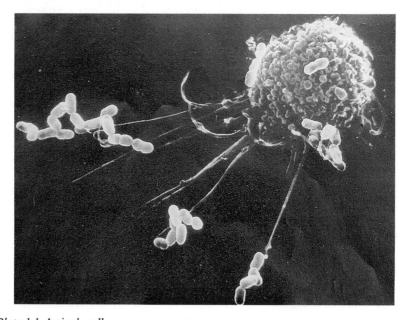

Plate 1.1 A single cell.

pattern; some tissues are composed of several cell types and others of a single cell type.

- Cells can move.
- Cells manufacture.
- Cells secrete and excrete.
- Cells can destroy.
- Each cell type has a lifespan; as they die they are replaced by an exact replica manufactured in one of the many body factories.

To illustrate a cell is almost impossible. Photographs make them appear flat! Try to picture a sea sponge which is a primitive structure composed of a group of similar cells (see Plates 1.1 and 1.2).

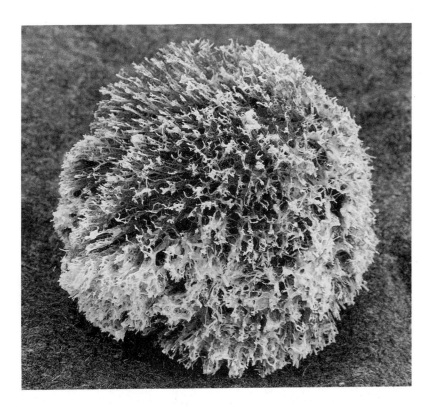

Plate 1.2 A sea sponge composed of a group of similar cells.

Bone

The bones provide a framework for other tissues to build on, and to encase and protect vital organs.

Bone is a dense connective tissue. Its structure is impregnated with bone salts (chiefly calcium carbonate and calcium phosphate). The outer shell of a bone is built in layers arranged in a concentric manner; this arrangement is called *compact bone*. Beneath the compact bone is a network or mesh arrangement; bone marrow fills the *medullary cavity* in the centre of a bone (see Plate 1.3).

Bone marrow is one of the body's factories, aiding in the production of cells. As well as acting as the body frame, bones are used as stores for mineral salts, thus they have several functions:

- They aid in the production of red blood cells.
- They store.
- They support.

Over the outermost layer of concentric bone lies the *periosteum* – a tough fibrous membrane. This is used by ligaments and muscles as a

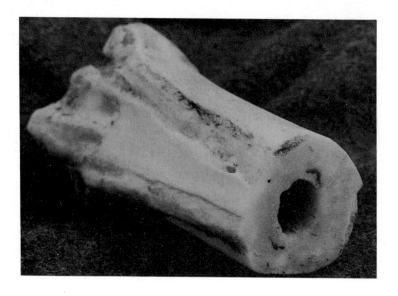

Plate 1.3 The medullary cavity. In life this contains bone marrow, the function of which is to manufacture cells.

means of attachment. It also feeds and nourishes the bone; for bone, just like all other tissue, requires constant rebuilding, feeding and cleansing. To achieve this a plexus of blood vessels is ingeniously incorporated around and within the structure; with a main artery entering each bone via a canal called the *nutrient foramen* (see Plate 1.4).

Joints

Joints are the point at which a bone surface designed to allow movement meets the similar surface of an adjoining bone. The opposing surfaces are covered with a tissue called *cartilage*. Cartilage is grey or white in appearance and semi-opaque. It is constructed so that it is capable of withstanding considerable pressure. Joints are enclosed by a capsule and the cavity created is filled with a lubricant liquid, *synovial fluid* (joint oil). The encapsulating membrane supports an inner layer of cells which manufacture and secrete the joint oil.

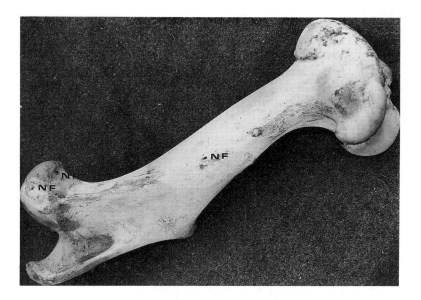

Plate 1.4 Nutrient foramina (NF) in the equine femur. Note the ridges on the bone caused by pull of attached muscles.

Ligaments

Ligaments span joints. They are flexible but not elastic as their role is to add strength and support to joints both internally (for example, the *ligamentum teres* of the hip and the *cruciate ligaments* of the stifle) and externally, where they limit the movement range of a joint to that which the shape of the opposing bone ends can comfortably sustain. A final role, not yet entirely understood, is that of their ability to assist in joint movement by loading with kinematic energy on stretch, then discharging the energy, thereby assisting the joint to return to its normal resting position.

Ligaments that are damaged are said to be *sprained*. The damage is usually the result of severe overstretching and it is almost impossible to correct such a situation as ligaments, unlike most other connective tissues, do not remodel to their original.

Muscles and tendons

The muscles that move the body and maintain the required posture against the forces of gravity are called *skeletal muscles*. They are dependent for effective function upon a nerve supply to command their actions. Their energy/fuel demands are very complex and are discussed in greater depth in Chapter 5.

Smooth muscle is found in the walls of blood vessels, the gut, the stomach and other internal organs. *Cardiac muscle* is specific to the heart.

Skeletal muscles pass over one or more joints. They are attached via the periosteum to the bone above and below the joint they are designed to influence. Muscles attached above the knees and hocks of the horse modify their structure as they near these joints, with their fibres becoming increasingly strong and compact, so that eventually the tissue resembles a hawser. This is called a *tendon*. Equine tendon examined microscopically demonstrates a crimp-like formation allowing for stretch and recoil when subjected to the intense demands created as the angle of pastern to ground at gallop is forced from approximately 45° to 90°.

Tendons have no mechanism to maintain an ambient central or core temperature. The heat within their core, generated by work at fast paces while the structure is being subjected to continual stretch and recoil, rapidly reaches a critical level. Any tissue becomes fragile at high temperature, thus the excessive rise in the core temperature of the working tendon contributes to tendon breakdown. Unfortunately tendons *never* regain their original characteristics following destruction, whatever the reason for the destruction.

The cardiovascular system (heart and blood vessels)

Blood circulates throughout the body infiltrating every single system and structure. It can be likened to a conveyor belt as it transports cells, oxygen, fuel, protective agents, repair kits and debris; in fact every component the body needs to sustain life, to cleanse, to repair and to protect itself.

The arterial system operates under high pressure. The pressure within its arterial vessels is achieved by the pumping action of the heart. The arterial blood is therefore able to act as an efficient delivery service. The blood in the veins is loaded with waste and debris, and conveys these to various waste disposal units. All waste is processed, with usable elements being recycled and the rest excreted in the form of urine, faeces, sweat and expelled gas; the latter exiting via the route through which air is inhaled, the trachea and nasal passages. Once the waste has been dumped the venous blood, which is under much less pressure than the arterial, returns to the heart, then to the lungs to be redirected for reloading.

The actual delivery of goods and the collection of waste takes place in tiny blood vessels called *capillaries*. The walls of the capillaries are specially designed to allow for the easy interchange of components, both to and from the various tissues and organs.

Blood has been called a *body barometer*. In the laboratory, tests have established a set of normal reference values for all the differing cells and substances found in blood. Variations from the accepted normal are studied to aid diagnosis if a problem has occurred, but the values can also be used as an indicator of the general health of a horse in the absence of problems.

Blood is part liquid, part cellular, with the cells suspended in the liquid *plasma*. There are different types of cells, and each family has a particular function.

● *Erythrocytes* are the red oxygen carrying cells.
● *Leucocytes* or white blood cells have several sub-divisions, each type having a specific role in the defence and repair mechanisms.

- *Platelets* are concerned with clotting. Damage to the wall of a blood vessel may allow blood to escape from the normally 'closed circuit' system; such blood loss which reduces the total volume is a disaster. In such an emergency the platelets activate and initiate chemical processes which convert liquid blood to a solid state, thus preventing escape.

Laboratory tests are used to build a blood picture. Blood for testing should be taken with the horse at rest (even minimal excitement changes the cell balance). As knowledge of the changes in blood chemistry and the behaviour of its components is subjected to increased research, blood taken pre- and post-exercise will allow values other than just cellular values to be scrutinized, and will assist in the assessment of other factors – tolerance to exercise, fitness level, and recovery after competition, being just a few examples.

Only vets are allowed to take blood from a horse. Laboratory technicians then prepare and test the blood, and the vet reads the test results and is able to report on the findings. A great number of tests are possible and while you (the owner) will be given a copy of the 'blood picture', the rows of names, abbreviations and figures will mean very little unless you have been trained to interpret the findings. For example, what do RBC and WBC mean (RBC = Red Blood Cells, WBC = White Blood Cells)? However, there are different types of white cells, all of which have their own accepted normal levels, and any deviation from the accepted 'normal' value is significant and to an expert is a vital piece in the jigsaw puzzle of diagnosis.

Table 1.1 gives a guide to the generally accepted 'normal' reference values of equine blood. It is not a full list of the possible biochemical estimations.

Table 1.1   Generally accepted normal reference values of equine blood.

	Thoroughbred	Non-Thoroughbred
red blood cells (RBC) $\times$ $10^{12}/1$	7.0 to 13.0	5.5 to 9.5
haemoglobin Hb/dl	10 to 18	8 to 14
white blood cells (WBC) $\times$ $10^9/1$	6 to 12	6 to 12
platelets $\times$ $10^9/1$	200 to 400	200 to 400
neutrophils $\times$ $10^9/1$	2.5 to 7.0	
lymphocytes $\times$ $10^9/1$	1.6 to 5.4	
monocytes $\times$ $10^9/1$	0.6 to 0.7	

Proteins – the total, the albumin and globulin levels – can be assessed, as can plasma fibrogen, urea, creatinine, and enzymes, one of which, creatinine kinase CPK, the three letters familiar to all, is associated with, among other conditions, muscle damage.

Blood values differ both in individuals and in breeds. It is the job of skilled personnel to analyse and report on the factual evidence supplied from the tested blood samples for conditions can be recognized by collating variance from the accepted normal 'picture'.

Lymphatic system

The body is composed largely of fluid which needs to be on the move constantly – to be *circulated*. The heart ensures that the cell-carrying blood is forced through arteries, capillaries and veins by means of the pressure created by the pumping action of the heart. Lymph, a fluid similar to blood plasma, contains proteins and other substances, all of which are needed by body components. It is found scattered throughout the entire structure, and is described as *tissue fluid* when not contained in lymph vessels.

The lymphatic system associates very closely with all veins, its maze of vessels lying alongside the veins. Filtering stations or clumps of *lymph nodes* are strategically sited within the network of lymphatic vessels. These lymph nodes help to combat infection and disease. If excessively activated by the presence of irritants they swell and become painful when palpated. All fluids from tissues which are not collected by the veins diffuse into the lymphatic vessels and slowly pass to a vessel called the *thoracic duct*. From there, via veins called the *innominate veins*, the fluids are returned to the main stream circulation.

The lymphatic system has no pressure pump to assist fluid movement; it is dependent to a large part on the variation of pressures within the tissues created by movement. Massage can be used to assist lymphatic flow.

Respiration

Oxygen is an essential ingredient. It combines chemically with body fuels, in particular with glucose, to provide the energy required for all metabolic processes.

Oxygen is absorbed into the blood within the lungs from the air drawn in through the upper respiratory tract. This consists of the nasal passages, the larynx, the pharynx and the trachea. The trachea sub-divides into two major bronchi, one for each lung. The bronchi divide and sub-divide, becoming smaller and smaller, until as the terminal bronchioles, they enter the air sacs or alveoli. The specialist walls of the alveoli allow the diffusion of gases both to and from the tiny blood vessels that enmesh their walls. Thus oxygen passes into the circulatory system.

Lack of oxygen dramatically reduces performance. Reduced oxygen delivery can be traced to many factors: upper airway disease is obviously one; the inability of the thoracic cage, within which the lungs are installed, to expand is another; irritant particles of dust can cause damage to the fragile walls of the air sacs, and such damage will stop the oxygen molecules passing through those walls for collection and then transport by red blood cells waiting in the capillaries enmeshing the walls of the air sacs.

The lungs are also utilized as a waste disposal unit to exhale unwanted gases and dissipate excess heat.

The respiratory and cardiovascular systems are inextricably linked by the body's need for oxygen. To ensure an adequate oxygen supply inbuilt safety mechanisms control the rate and depth of respiration along with the rate at which the heart beats, but these safety mechanisms are useless if the flow of air from the exterior is reduced or curtailed. Fatigue occurs early in the absence of oxygen.

Nervous system

The various components of the nervous system master-mind communication, recording, analysis and action following analysis, control of all systems, control of movement, control of the heart, response to pain, to stimuli, control of temperature ... the list is infinite.

Central nervous system
The central nervous system consists of the brain and spinal cord. For maximum protection these are housed within cavities surrounded by bone – the brain within the skull and the spinal cord within the vertebral column. Both brain and spinal cord are wrapped in three layers of protective tissue and suspended in fluid. Specialist *cranial nerves* arise directly from the brain and leave the skull, each via its own

aperture. In the horse there are 12 pairs. These nerves control highly specialized functions such as smell, sight and hearing.

Destruction of, compression to, disease within, or any disturbance to the normal function of central nervous tissue is irreversible and creates havoc.

Peripheral nervous system

At the intersection between the bones of the vertebral column, a pair of *spinal nerves* arise from the spinal cord. These nerves are in continual communication with the spinal cord and via it, with the brain. The nerves pass outward into the body mass, elongating and sub-dividing as they go, enmeshing the entire structure within an elaborate control network.

Disturbance to nervous tissues lying outside the central complex effectively cuts communication to and from all the structures serviced by the nerve or nerves involved; muscle tissue is unable to function in the absence of signals from its *motor nerve* – it is paralysed. Normally recorded sensations, such as heat, cold, pain or position in space are not appreciated; the circulation within the affected area is impaired and the skin cannot react normally to external stimuli.

The nervous system is the first to be developed in the growing fetus. At birth the foal arrives with several brain co-ordinated actions; it can stand, suck and smell, and from the moment of birth an incredible learning process takes place. Repeated actions are logged in the brain, the messages invoked by the actions having been passed by nerves in the tissues to the spinal cord and then to the brain. *Logged actions become accepted as normal, thus if a foal is always led with its head turned toward the handler the brain will accept this as the norm.*

Schooling or teaching requires care. A signal is given by the rider, and the horse responds by moving, turning or halting. The rider must choose a separate signal for each movement. If the signals are repeated often enough the horse's brain logs them and it will respond by performing the movement it has learnt as the correct response. Confusion arises if the horse is given an incorrect or indecisive signal. The brain does not know how to react and the horse fails to produce the movement required by the rider. Some horses learn faster than others – clarity and exact repetition of command are essential; punishment causes confusion.

Damage to central nervous tissue rarely recovers; damage to nerves outside the central part of the system normally resolves with partial or complete recovery occurring. Recovery can be enhanced by therapy.

Digestive system

The digestive system refines and processes all the substances the horse eats. Just like any factory, the body needs raw ingredients to sustain production. A factory usually has the required raw materials delivered ready prepared for immediate use, but the horse's body does not. It needs to process its food, and chewing is the first stage of refinement. This is essential to activate digestive activities. Pulverizing plant matter uses energy, as does the refining and selection of the necessary ingredients: the nutrients, proteins, carbohydrates, fats, minerals, vitamins and water. Energy is wasted if a diet is badly balanced, too dry, hard to break down, or if it has insufficient bulk. It is also wasted if the horse is unable to chew correctly because of teeth problems.

Digestion within the stomach and intestines is aided by secretions manufactured in the liver, spleen and pancreas. These organs are also able to store nutrients for future use.

The digestive process started in the mouth, continues, with extraction of useful ingredients, throughout the intestines until the waste is compacted and expelled as droppings. The quality of the droppings should be noted. If they are too dry, too sloppy, sour-smelling, if they contain unchewed or undigested food, or any other abnormality this can indicate digestive failure.

The intestines are a canal which starts in the mouth and ends at the anus. The canal is not truly part of the internal architecture of the body as is, for example, the liver. It is a very lengthy convoluted tube contiguous with the body's outer surface. This design prevents any toxic material entering the abdominal cavity should something poisonous be eaten or inadvertently created. The intestines move continuously with a wave-like ripple, shifting their contents in a continuous unidirectional flow from stomach to anus.

The kidneys and bladder

The kidneys are not merely organs of excretion, they are essential for the maintenance of the correct acid-based balance of the blood and tissue fluids. They also conserve metabolic products and have the ability to convert back into usable assets substances being excreted as waste.

After filtration within the kidneys the unwanted liquid and unessential chemicals (*urine*) pass down the urethra to the bladder, from where, when sufficient is collected, it is voided to the exterior. The colour, texture and smell of the urine are important. It should be clear and odourless.

Summary

This has been a very brief description of the body systems. To summarise:

- The frame is bone.
- Muscles move the frame as commanded by the nervous system.
- The nervous system also controls and commands the balanced interlinking of the functions of all the systems which deal with delivery, disposal, feeding, building, defending, seeing, smelling,

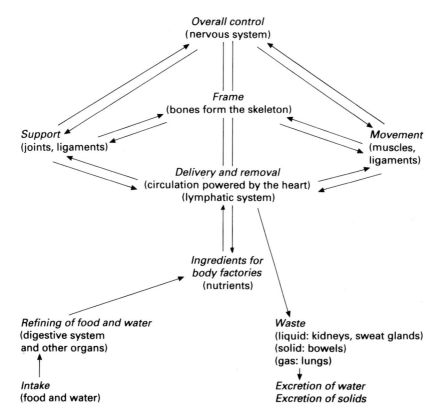

Fig. 1.1 Interrelationship of the body's systems.

responding, keeping warm, resting, moving, excreting and breathing ... everything.

The body functions as a whole, and those who try to influence its systematic activities, be it in health or disease, must try to comprehend this very important fact. Everything from the smallest cell to the largest organ, from the visual image we call a horse to its response to its human master, every feature of its make-up is inextricably inter-connected and it can only function if all the systems not only work, but are also maintained in a healthy condition by having all the necessary ingredients freely available in the correct balanced proportions.

2 Nutrition: Herbs, Their Benefits, including sources of Vitamins and Minerals

Herbs and Their Benefits

There is no need to debate or even question the fact that the planet on which we live is fully stocked to cater for all our needs. Unfortunately, we have either become too lazy or forgotten how to seek, grow, prepare and use these natural goods. Synthetic substitutes, invented by man, have no natural planetary niche and today we face problems which could not have occurred naturally and for which we have no solutions. Chemicals need more chemicals to destroy them; they are not biologically degradable. Such synthetic substances are alien to planetary ecology, there is no mode of recycling as with the natural substances utilized in the 'pre-pollution' era.

Permaculture

The word *permaculture* is derived from the term 'permanent agriculture', denoting a self-sustaining agricultural system. The science of agriculture, the means by which essential raw materials for the perpetuation of life in all species are provided, is of paramount importance. We require a multi-crop of vegetation which must include annual and perennial plants, mineral rich soil, water, air and animals. The plants, including the trees, must complement each other's growth requirements and be appropriate for both the soil and climatic conditions of the growing area, be it garden or pasture.

One of the most interesting features when regarding nutrition as a whole, is that only *very small* amounts of trace elements and vitamins are needed by the living body, provided they are obtained from natural sources.

Herbs

Herbs are plants. They contain nutrients required by other life forms. The Romans introduced around 400 species of herbs to northern Europe, but the knowledge of their attributes and properties, both medicinal and for the general maintenance of general health, stretches back thousands of years. There is evidence of a *Herbal* composed in China around 2700 BC, and medical prescriptions were in use and recorded in writing in Egypt around 1800 BC. Even though minerals are mentioned in these writings, $5/6$ of the recommended ingredients are herbal in origin. The lore of plant gathering, growing, preserving and the use of roots followed complex rituals handed down from family member to family member. This tradition still survives in remote areas and when searching for genuine herbal information I have often been told that the present 'healer' learnt the secrets from 'her pa' who 'had it from his ma' and so on, with five or six past generations often quoted.

Medicine

To most of us 'medicine' means the science of healing *after* catastrophe. The dictionary states 'medicine is the science or practice of the *prevention* of disease; also of non-surgical methods of treatment following a diagnosed problem'.

Health

Prevention rather than cure is the message of herbalists. The use of herbs is therefore primarily aimed at promoting total health. What do we mean by health? It is a state in which an entire cellular mass, combined to form a recognisable named species, is in a state of harmony, with:

- all the necessary ingredients present,
- all the storage chambers filled,
- all the internal organs complementing each other's activities,
- all the systems running smoothly,
- the blood and oxygen correctly balanced,

- the body mass fuelled to meet the demands of a workload deter-mined by the level of daily activity, and
- the fluid levels and acid-base balance accurate for the species.

To achieve and maintain this state imposes a need to continually rebuild, replenish and restore. These activities demand the availability of easily assimilated nutrients. Those from natural sources require the expenditure of less body energy to refine, synthesize and extract the required minerals/vitamins/salts, than do the man-made chemical substitutes, most of which have unwanted often detrimental, side effects.

Additives

The horseman of today is bombarded with new products claiming to make the horse 'go faster', 'grow hoof', 'shine coat', 'avoid fatigue' and 'perform better'. There are 'feed mixes', 'feed supplements' and 'feed additives', all of which extol their own particular virtues. After all, the power of advertizing is subtle one-upmanship! Stand back and consider before more money goes in at one end of your horse and comes out at the other. How *can* an additive 'reduce oxygen requirements'? It is a scientific impossibility!

Feeding

Ideally stabled horses should be pastured daily, preferably on an old ley surrounded by natural hedges, forming an environment rich in different plants. Horses have not yet lost their natural ability to choose plants containing the vitamins and minerals which instinctively they appreciate they lack. They will help themselves, not gorging but lipping a leaf off this, a stem off that – remember minute amounts rebalance systems. To bake a successful cake you need the correct balance of ingredients; an excess of one or reduction of another results in failure. The body is no different and problems arise if additives are incorrectly balanced, over-supplementation of one mineral preventing the utilization of another. For example the absorption of calcium and copper can be inhibited by zinc if over supplementation occurs.

Herbs balance requirements naturally if they are freely available, but they need to be grown in a permaculture situation so they can scavenge their requirements from the soil. If the soil lacks the necessary nutrients, the plants will not contain the substances accredited to their species in the descriptive literature Accounts extolling the benefits of each variety of herb assume the herb was grown under ideal conditions; ideal in that the plant was able to draw freely from the growth area all the ingredients required to synthesize the products for which it is renowned. Some species store nutrients in their root structure, some in their leaves and some in their stems.

Before rushing into designing and planting a herb garden it is sensible to have your soil analysed, then to study the needs of your horse, taking into account workload, season, age and breed. Each of these facets will modify the intake requirement, and as it is exceptionally difficult to achieve the correct balance, it is preferable to allow natural selection by the animal, particularly as most herbs are not 'single suppliers'. For instance garlic (which grows wild) is a source of antibacterial substances and vitamins A, B_1, B_2 and C. The onion is rich in vitamins A, B_1, B_2, C and E. Chives, a cousin of both garlic and the onion, are easy to grow and a few chopped are not unpalatable.

The ability of the horse to 'doctor' itself is well illustrated by the fact that known 'bleeders' will, if the plants are available, eat plantains, a herb used for haemorrhage control in human herbal remedies.

To change from a 'prepared' feed, which supposedly contains all the essentials, and to search for, and feed a balanced diet meeting all requirements using plants obtained from nature is very time-consuming. Unfortunately natural supplementation is an 'all or nothing regime'. It cannot be a half and half situation, for if you supplement by allowing your horse to graze and then add artificial supplements 'in case factor X is missing' you are more likely to create problems than to reduce them.

Nutrition

Nutritional experts can only be expected to offer guidelines. It is quite impossible to generalize a feed programme as each animal, just as each human, has characteristics common to its genetic background.

For the average horse the essential requirements are a balance containing:

- Water
- Protein

- Carbohydrate
- Fat
- Minerals
- Vitamins

Functions of the nutrients

Water
Water is essential for all metabolic processes. A water deficiency is very serious and even though the daily intake will vary, a horse needs access to fresh water at all times. Water is lost:

- During the excretion of urine
- In the faeces
- When sweating
- Via respiratory evaporation during expiration.

The amount of dry matter fed will also influence the daily water requirements.

Protein
Amino acids, some of which are synthesized by the body, while others are obtained from external sources, constitute the fundamental structure of all proteins. Proteins form the structural material of the tissues, the muscles and the body organs, and they are important regulators of function, in common with enzymes and hormones.

Excess protein which is not structurally required, can be converted into glucose to be stored and utilized as energy. However an excessive protein intake is *not* beneficial. Its side effects include loss of speed and early fatigue.

Carbohydrate
The primary source of energy in equine diet is culled from the carbohydrate intake. This energy is absorbed from the intestine as glucose, and any excess which is not immediately required, is stored as glycogen both in muscle and in the liver. The muscle store is ready for immediate use on demand, during exercise and that stored in the liver is available as a 'back up' to be released into the blood stream where it is rapidly transported to areas of need.

The correct level of glucose is controlled by insulin. An excess intake of carbohydrate can cause the blood glucose level to rise too rapidly with the consequence of an increased insulin response which may promote a temporary 'rebound' (*hypoglycaemia*). This may show as inco-ordination and sweating. Thus sudden carbohydrate loading must be carefully monitored.

Fat

Horses utilize fats as an energy source during prolonged aerobic muscle work. Fat is mainly stored in adipose tissue. Fats are a highly concentrated source of energy able to supply twice the number of calories, weight for weight, as compared with carbohydrates. The exercise demands must be assessed prior to increasing the fat ration as fats are *not* a substitute for carbohydrate. The feeding of 5–15% of acceptable fats as a source of dietary energy is a reasonable level. Corn oil is one source of acceptable fat.

Minerals

Minerals are inorganic elements processed in the main via plants which when ingested deliver the minerals they carry to their host. Minerals are essential ingredients for health. Calcium, phosphorus, potassium, sodium, chloride, magnesium and sulphur are all required in reasonable amounts. Iron, copper, cobalt, iodine, manganese and zinc are needed in lesser amounts, with only minute amounts of selenium required. This list is compiled from 1993 reports; as research continues other trace elements will undoubtedly be added.

Minerals are involved in

- Energy transfer
- Fluid balance
- Maintenance of osmotic pressure
- Activity within both the nervous and muscular systems
- They also assist in forming many of the body structures

Mineral loss

Horses loose minerals (*electrolytes*) in significant amounts in sweat. Some, for example, sodium potassium and sodium chloride, must be replaced following loss either by an electrolyte supplement in water if the horse will drink, or by drenching if it will not, or, in cases of extreme exhaustion, by using a saline drip. Excessive supplementation pre-exercise is of little use for two reasons. First, the body always maintains a balance applicable to its immediate situation – at rest in a stall, pastured or in a normal daily exercise routine the requirements are low and any surfeit fed is excreted in the urine; second, indiscriminate loading has a tendency to interfere with normal absorption, thus some minerals, even though present become 'locked up' and unavailable.

Vitamins

Vitamins are complex organic compounds, micronutrients, which are essential for health. Some are manufactured by the body but once again plants supply the majority. Plant tissue manufactures vitamins during its growing cycle, and different plants or 'herbage' supply variable quantities and categories.

Vitamins are sub-divided into two groups: those classified as *water soluble* and those classified as *fat soluble*. For successful reactivity many vitamins need to interact with one or more minerals. Vitamins were first recognized in 1911 and by 1977 fifteen had been 'discovered'. *The Dictionary of Vitamins* (1984 edition) lists 23 and there are undoubtedly many more as yet unidentified, but certainly present, probably both organically and within the body components. Vitamins are involved in:

- Tissue building
- Body defence
- Digestion
- Food assimilation
- All manufacturing processes
- Nerve conductivity
- All metabolic processes

Lack of vitamins or an incorrect balance gives rise to conditions classed as deficiency diseases. Beriberi (caused by vitamin B deficiency) was described as early as 2600 BC in China. No 'cure' was 'found', or certainly not recorded, until 1880 – nearly 5000 years later. A reduction in the incidence of the disease was noticed when Takaki stopped using highly milled (polished) rice on board Japanese naval ships. Polishing the rice removes the outer thiamine rich (vitamin B) covering or 'coat' of the grains. This example also serves to illustrate how carefully nutritious intake must be handled.

Preference for natural sources is obvious – the body has developed and evolved side by side with the environment and all elements within its structure are naturally adapted to assimilate plant-produced nutrients. Body components do not easily recognize synthetic products and are often unable to utilize or ingest them, with many merely excreted having been classified as 'incompatible'.

As stated earlier, natural herbage and grains contain most vitamins, but the herbage must be of good quality. Bleached hay, hay with serious leaf loss, poor quality, stale or mouldy food will all have had their original vitamin content depleted. Horses fed poor quality forage and who do not have access to pasture and sunlight will require vitamin supplementation, not only in their food, but also by the use of ultraviolet light in a solarium to enable the horse to synthesise vitamin D. Vitamin D is involved in the metabolism of calcium which is essential not only for bone structure but also for efficient muscle activity. Thus a lack of natural sunlight is serious and horses who suffer this will not be as healthy as those exposed to natural sunlight. In these instances a solarium will go some way to improving health. Each animal should be considered individually and a ration both balanced and appropriate to its needs formulated.

Herbs
Unfortunately, the many changes in the agricultural policies have led to the destruction of 'natural' meadows where a variety of differing species supported each other. The indiscriminate use of nitrogen has caused massive changes in soil composition and many areas have become practically sterile as intensive cropping has robbed the soil of all components. However it is perfectly possible to sow and grow many of the common herbs. Make certain the soil is in good heart before planting or sowing. Seaweed is an excellent compound for putting life back into the soil in denuded areas.

It is possible to purchase dried herbs and herb mixes. The bulk amount required will vary, because there is some loss of content when herbs are provided chopped and dried rather than being offered fresh. If you 'gather' allow for a loss of 30% of potency. This loss occurs within 24 to 36 hours of gathering. Herbs must be dried correctly and always stored in a cool dry area.

Taste can be an indicator of use: pleasant tasting herbs are tonic herbs and help maintain health; medical herbs tend to be bitter – not all are edible, some are poisonous, or if their leaves are safe their roots are not. Herbalism is a science – to become proficient requires indepth study.

'There are no known side effects from herbs used knowledgeably and wisely. *Knowledge* and *wisdom* are the key words. Herbs cannot be used indiscriminately without knowledge, no more than can food. We must use common sense, fortified with a basic knowledge of the properties of herbs and an appreciation of body requirements in order to use them effectively.'

(Stan Malstrom, *Own Your Own Body*)

The first part of this section has mentioned the bare nutritional requirements of a horse and touches on a very few of the complex interactions and processes involved in the functions of living. This section endeavours to expand the theme by linking vitamins and mineral necessities to herb sources in rather more depth. The herbs discussed are not confined to those found in the UK alone. Vitamins and minerals are described, their role in body metabolism is suggested, herb sources are recorded and possible deficiency characteristics suggested.

It must be realized that deficiency conditions result from multiple influences, rather than from a single factor.

The term *metabolism* refers to the highly complex and complicated changes the body cells, in their various factory systems, achieve using the ingredients delivered to the digestive system in the shape of ingested food. Some of the changes occur as a result of activity by resident intestinal microbial elements, some by enzyme activity, some by interaction with cell secretions, some by coupling with minerals, and some by complex chemical reactions.

You will notice that no values are given in some sections of the text headed 'Equine Requirements'. This is because exact values have *not* been established, *but* it is appreciated that horses do need all the vitamins and minerals listed.

Once again it is obvious from the herb sources mentioned that the free ranging animal would have been able to select herbage containing the mineral/vitamin components necessary to sustain life.

Sunlight

Before considering the herbal sources of the nutrients required, it is essential to consider in more depth a freely available essential health constituent which has already been mentioned in passing: i.e. *sunlight*. As with many notable scientific discoveries the power and necessity of sunlight for health was an accidental discovery. Dr John Ott is a photographer, his speciality being time-lapse photography. Suffice it to say that after many years of experimenting he realized some light rays essential for the full growth and fertility of the plants he was photographing were being filtered out by the glass that protected the plants, so he turned to assessing the effects on laboratory animals of lack of light, and exposure to varying light wave lengths. Slowly he came to realize that the full spectrum of daylight was essential for harmonious living.

Much has been written about the nutritional requirements of animals and humans. The complex role played by natural minerals and vitamins is slowly being unravelled but the need for one vital commodity is rarely, if ever, mentioned – that commodity is *sunlight*.

All energy is derived in some manner from the sun. Consider plants which *photosynthesize* or absorb sunlight to create the energy they require to live, grow and reproduce. The green colour of the plant arises from chlorophyll. Molecules of chlorophyll are able to absorb sunlight and in a complex chain reaction, combine with water and carbon dioxide to create carbohydrates – the 'food' from which the plant derives the energy for its complex life pattern. During the conversion of absorbed sunlight into carbohydrate, oxygen is created and released to the atmosphere. Some species of plant, their seeds or fruit are eventually eaten by members of the animal kingdom. The consumer's body extracts the nutrients it requires and slowly, a complex cycle (Kreb's cycle) breaks down the carbohydrate content, extracting energy and utilizing that energy as and where it is pertinent and required from each step of Kreb's cycle. The process eventually reforms the original water and carbon dioxide, both of which are excreted in re-usable forms thereby completing the 'natural cycle'.

Plants and animals have co-existed since animal life initially evolved. The sun was here first, then plants developed, followed by the animal kingdom. Today, in the twentieth century, life is very different: we shut ourselves from the sun and have even become fearful of its effect upon us. Unfortunately it is the way we use the sun rather than the sun itself which does the harm. Gentle exposure encourages the production of the chemical melanin which darkens the skin and gives protection from the damaging rays. The world's populace adapted to climatic conditions, with dark-skinned people near the equator and light-skinned people away from the equator. Dark skins filter out damaging rays and light skins allow absorption in areas where the sunlight is less strong.

There are shade-loving plants, plants who prefer light from the north and full sun lovers; site a plant in a situation for which it is not suited and it is unlikely to thrive; overexposure is as harmful as under-exposure.

In today's world many domestic animals spend more and more time indoors screened from sunlight. Boxes may be in a barn, shaded by an overhang, grills on doors prevent the animal putting its head outside its box and many horses spend as much as 23 hours out of every 24 in their boxes. Even those turned out wear screening New Zealand rugs. They are being starved of an ingredient vital for the metabolic activities of calcium and phosphorus – the correct absorption in the intestine, retention and mobilization. No matter if the formulated diet contains calcium and phosphorus in the assumed correct ratio, unless the 'sunshine vitamin' (vitamin D) is present problems are inevitable.

How does an animal get vitamin D? Unfortunately the distribution of vitamin D in herbage is poor. Some is formed when certain pasture species begin to fade provided they are exposed to sunlight at the time. The ideal time for that exposure is the two hours either side of midday – early morning sun or late afternoon sun will have less effect. Lack of natural vitamin D presupposes the Prototype Designer did not consider an era when sunlight would be in short supply, for the body manufactures D in response to exposure to sunlight.

Life requires many things to sustain it. Down the millennia different species have adapted to their native environmental conditions. They may be smaller if they have less sun but nevertheless they have adapted. Problems begin when species are moved to different environmental conditions, particularly if these movements occur at critical developmental stages in the animal's life. Air travel has made the transportation of the horse a commonplace event. Consider such a journey: an animal roams the pastures in New Zealand at a formative phase of its development. It is utilizing a wide range of mineral and vitamin rich herbage and natural water in its development and it has hours of sunlight filtering through an atmosphere free from the UK levels of pollution. The animal is suddenly switched, over a 36 hour period, to the UK. It is probably stabled on arrival and therefore *cut off from sunlight*. The feed and water bear no resemblance to those to which its body's metabolic processes are accustomed. If it is an infoal mare, how can the growing fetus be unaffected by such a catastrophic change?

Abrams in 1978 pointed out that many horses are exercised in the early morning before being housed for the rest of the day, and thus must be lacking essential sunlight.

A problem with any deficiency is that rarely is it immediately apparent. Lack of nutrients in one generation will be rectified by the extraction of the necessary nutrients from the body's stores. Breed from that animal and the next generation will be a shade less robust. The spiral will continue downward until problems such as porous bones, spontaneous fractures, or reduced muscle activity become agonizingly apparent.

If possible, include natural sunlight in your horse's diet – after all, it is a free additive! If a solarium is to be substituted as the source of light, check the bulbs – they must emit full spectrum light to be of value.

For the readers who are busy thinking 'sun exposure equals skin cancer', *please* substitute '*sunburn* or *skinfry* equals damage'. Traumatize skin and it will react unfavourably. It also follows that an excess, no matter in what context, is bad for any living species. The human race tends to overindulge; animals and plants take what they need. Animals will move out of excess sunlight into shade if it is available and plants operate shut down mechanisms to protect themselves. Solarium manufacturers should indicate minimum and maximum graded time exposures. *Do not* be tempted to overexpose on the principle that if five minutes is good ten minutes will be better. If your horse is not used to exposure it will take time to adapt.

Historical uses for herbs

Herbs have been used for many different reasons down the ages. Listed below are some of their key purposes.

Alternative – Herbs used to change existing nutritious and elimination processes to regulate body functions.

Analgesic – Herbs used to ease pain when taken internally.

Anodyne – Herbs used to ease pain when used externally.

Antibiotic – Herbs used to terminate growth of harmful micro-organisms.

Antihydropic – Herbs used to eliminate excess body fluid.

Anti-inflammatory –Herbs used to reduce inflammation.

Antipyretic – Herbs used to relieve fevers.

Antiseptic – Herbs used to stop, fight and counteract toxic bacteria.

Antispasmodic – Herbs used to sooth contractions or coughing.

Antisyphilitic – Herbs used to relieve venereal diseases.

Aphrodisiac – Herbs used to cure problems of impotency and restore sexual power.

Aromatic – Herbs that have an aromatic taste and stimulate the mucous membrane in the intestines.

Astringent – Herbs used to condense tissues and stop discharges.

Calmative – Herbs used to calm the nervous system.

Cardiac – Herbs used to make the heart stronger.

Carminative – Herbs used to eliminate gas from the digestive system.

Cathartic – Herbs used to encourage purging from the bowel.

Cell proliferant – Herbs used to heal and stimulate new cell growth.

Cholagogue – Herbs to increase flow of bile into the duodenum.

Demulcent – Herbs used to soothe and protect areas which are painful or inflamed internally.

Depurant – Herbs used to purify the blood, stimulating the elimination procedures.

Diaphoretic – Herbs used to encourage perspiration.

Digestant – Herbs containing enzymes, amino acids, etc., to help in the digestion of food.

Diuretic – Herb used to increase urine flow.

Emmenagogue – Herbs used to stimulate suppressed menstrual flow.

Emolient – Herbs used to soften and protect the skin.

Expectorant – Herbs used to eliminate toxic mucus from the respiratory system.

Febrifuge – Herbs used to reduce fevers.

Hemostatic – Herbs used to stop bleeding.

Hepatic – Herbs used to strengthen the liver and increase the flow of bile.

Hormonal – Herbs containing hormonal properties.

Laxative – Herbs used as a mild laxative, stimulating bile and secretions rather than irritating the bowel.

Mucilaginous – Herbs with an adhering, expanding property, with soothing qualities for healing.

Nervine – Herbs used to calm the nerves.

Nutritive – Herbs that are nutritious and encourage growth.

Purgative – Herbs used to cause purging from the bowels, used generally in a combination with other herbs to control action.

Relaxant or *Sedative* – Herbs used for their calming properties.

Stimulant – Herbs used to increase the energy levels of the body, or its parts or organs.

Stomachic – Herbs used to strengthen the stomach and encourage the appetite.

Sudorific – Herbs that encourage perspiration.
Tonic – Herbs that stimulate and give the body energy.
Vermicide – Herbs used to kill parasites.
Vermufuge – Herbs used to expel worms.
Vulnerary – Herbs that encourage the healing of wounds.

Vitamins and Their Herb Sources

All books on equine nutrition list vitamins as an essential requirement. Most include at least short sections on vitamins A, the B family, C, D and E. However we are still a long way from a full list and exact requirement values are mostly unknown. On pages 39–42 you will find information on vitamins H, K, P and U, together with PABA. These have been included *not* because they appear in equine nutritional literature, but because they are present in the *natural herbage* that grows where wild horses lived and therefore must have formed part of their diet. References to herb sources pinpoint alfalfa as the most common denominator, with dandelion not far behind. 'Alfalfa hay', I can hear the cry, but remember it will have had its vitamin content edited *very considerably* by drying, crushing and in leaf loss. It can be grown and fed fresh, and if fertilized with a seaweed preparation, it should contain all its vitamins and minerals (see the section on Minerals and Their Herb Sources).

This text cannot be construed as dictating proven and definite values. The suggested equine requirements have been taken from the tables published in the United States and *Canadian Tables of Feed Composition*. Values are expressed in units per kilogram of diet, 100% dry basis.

N.B.: It must be noted that as research continues the values expressed here *may* change. If an animal is allowed free range, free selection and the appropriate herbage is present with the essential nutrients in the soil, the animal will balance its own required intake.

Vitamin A (Retinol)
Fat soluble. Essential for the body to manufacture visual purple (*rhodopsin*), which is necessary for night vision.

Vitamin A requires fats as well as minerals to be assimilated. It is an antioxidant. Antioxidants protect other substances from uncontrolled oxidations that damage cells. They help keep pollutants in check. (Antioxidants are vitamins A, C, E and selenium.)

Equine requirements:

Working animal	1600	i.u./kg
Pregnant mare	3400	i.u./kg
Lactating mare	2800	i.u./kg
Young stock	2000	i.u./kg

Associated with:
Vision
Maintenance of normal epithelium. (The epithelium lines and protects many body organs including the respiratory and digestive tracts.)
Healthy skin
Reproduction
Bone development
Cartilage integrity
Immune responses to disease including respiratory disease

Main signs of deficiency:
Eye disorders
Dry brittle coat
Susceptibility to infection
Defective bone modelling

Herb Sources

Alfalfa	Fenugreek	Peppermint
Burdock	Garlic	Pike
Capsicum	Ginger	Red clover
Catnip	Ginseng	Red raspberry
Camomile	Goldenseal	Rose hips
Comfrey	Kelp	Rosemary
Dandelion	Marshmallow	Sage
Eyebright	Mullein	Yarrow
Fennel	Papaya	Yellow dock

Vitamin B₁ (Thiamine)

Vitamin B_1 (Thiamine)

Water soluble. Also called morale or pep vitamins. All B vitamins should be taken as a B complex, i.e. one B alone is useless.

Equine requirements:

Young stock	3.0 mg/kg
Others	Unknown

Associated with:
Protein and carbohydrate metabolism (Krebs' cycle)
Digestion
Maintenance of normal red blood count
Muscle tone of heart, intestines and stomach

Main signs of deficiency:
Loss of mental alertness
Loss of appetite
Respiratory problems
Heart irregularities
Fatigue

Herb sources

Alfalfa	Dandelion	Hops
Blue Cohosh	Eyebright	Kelp
Burdock	Fenugreek	Licorice
Capsicum	Garlic	Marshmallow
Cascara	Ginger	Mullein
Catnip	Goldenseal	Papaya
Chickweed	Hawthorn	Red clover

Vitamin B$_2$ (Riboflavin)

Water soluble. Vitamin B$_2$ is not destroyed by heat, oxidation or acid. There is increased need during stress.

Equine requirements:

Adult maintenance requirement	2.2 mg/kg
Others	Unknown

Associated with:
Healthy skin, coat, hooves
Absorption of iron
Utilization of carbohydrates, fat protein

Main signs of deficiency:
Digestive disturbances
Anaemia
Fatigue
Poor growth
Severe weight loss

Herb Sources

Alfalfa	Dandelion	Hops
Blue cohosh	Eyebright	Kelp
Capsicum	Fenugreek	Licorice
Cascara	Ginger	Marshmallow
Catnip	Goldenseal	Mullein
Chickweed	Hawthorn	Papaya
		Red clover

Vitamin B₃ (Niacin or Nicotinic Acid, Nicotinamide)

Water soluble. The body can manufacture its own niacin.

Equine requirements:
Unknown; produced by the animal as required?

Associated with:
Nervous system function
Circulation of blood
Metabolism of proteins, carbohydrates, fats
Cell respiration

Main signs of deficiency can include:
Severe digestive problems

Herb Sources

Alfalfa	Eyebright	Licorice
Blue cohosh	Fenugreek	Marshmallow
Burdock	Ginger	Mullein
Capsicum	Goldenseal	Papaya
Catnip	Hawthorn	Red clover
Chickweed	Hops	Rose hips
Dandelion	Kelp	

Vitamin B₅ (Pantothenic Acid)

Water soluble. It is found in all living cells. It is known as the anti-stress vitamin, and can be produced by naturally occurring bacteria in the intestines.

Equine requirements:
Unknown; produced by the animal as required?

Associated with:
Auto-immune system building antibodies
The metabolism of protein, carbohydrate fats

Wound healing
Avoidance of fatigue
Drug detoxification
Chemical transmitted at the synapse of nerve

Main signs of deficiency:
Unknown

Herb Sources

Alfalfa	Chickweed	Hops
Black cohosh	Dandelion	Horsetail
Blue cohosh	Eyebright	Kelp
Burdock	Fenugreek	Licorice
Capsicum	Ginger	Marshmallow
Cascara	Goldenseal	Mullein
Catnip	Hawthorn	Papaya
		Red clover

Vitamin B$_6$ (Pyridoxamine)

Water soluble, it is excreted within eight hours of ingestion. Higher amounts are needed during pregnancy and lactation, and with high protein diets.

Equine requirements:
Unknown; produced by the animal as required?

Associated with:
Production of antibodies
DNA and RNA synthesis
Haemoglobin synthesis
Magnesium assimilation
Helps to metabolize fats, carbohydrates and protein
Aids in absorption of B$_{12}$
Body fluid balance by regulating potassium and sodium levels in the body

Main signs of deficiency:
No information available. Possibly muscle malfunction.
Braunlich (1974) suggested horses undergoing intensive training and fed high protein levels need B$_6$ supplementation.

Natural sources:
Carrots, Molasses, Wheat bran

Herb Sources

Alfalfa	Dandelion	Kelp
Blue cohosh	Eyebright	Licorice
Burdock	Fenugreek	Marshmallow
Capsicum	Ginger	Mullein
Cascara	Goldenseal	Papaya
Catnip	Hawthorn	Red clover
Chickweed	Hops	

Vitamin B₉ (Folicin or Folic Acid)

Water soluble. Folic acid was named because it is present in the 'foliage' of certain plants. Also considered to be the 'other anti-anaemia vitamin'.

Equine requirements:
Adult: considered to be 20 mg/day but no established levels

Associated with:
Synthesis of DNA and RNA
Transmission of genetic code
Associates with B_{12} to prevent anaemia
Disease resistance

Main signs of deficiency:
Poor performance
Anaemia

Natural sources:
Root vegetables

Herb Sources

Alfalfa	Dandelion	Kelp
Blue cohosh	Eyebright	Licorice
Burdock	Fenugreek	Marshmallow
Capsicum	Ginger	Mullein
Cascara	Goldenseal	Papaya
Catnip	Hawthorn	Red clover
Chickweed	Hops	

Vitamin B₁₂ (Cobalamin)

Water soluble. It is called the red vitamin. Unlike most water soluble vitamins it can be stored by the body.

Equine requirements:
Unknown; produced by the animal as required (microbial synthesis)?
Vitamin B_{12} deficiency is considered to be secondary to a deficiency of
  cobalt.

Associated with:
Essential for all basic metabolic processes
Excess of dietary protein increases the need for B_{12}
Increased performance levels increases the need for B_{12}

Main signs of deficiency:
Anaemia
Lack of metabolic activity

N.B.: The identification, B_{12}, is considered by experts in nutrition to
represent not one, but rather a complex group of compounds. These
compounds are involved in nearly every cell activity and metabolic
process.
If B_{12} is lacking, supplementation may need to be by injection. The
body may be unable to absorb B_{12} in cases of deficiency and there are
no known vegetation sources.

Natural sources; Herb sources
None

Vitamin C (Ascorbic acid)
Water soluble. The first vitamin discovered by man, it is a cure for
scurvy. It needs to be replaced daily; most animals manufacture their
own vitamin C. It is an antioxidant and a universal antitoxin, which
means it helps protect against harmful oxidation that damages cells,
and protects against poisonous and harmful substances of all kinds. It
has a primary role in the formation of collagen and helps the body's
absorption of iron.

Equine requirements:
No established levels
Manufactured by animal

Associated with:
Collagen synthesis in all tissues
Interlinks with B_{12}
Defence against the invasion of the body by bacterial and viral inci-
  dents

Improved wound healing
Iron metabolism

Main signs of deficiency:
Disturbed collagen metabolism in young animals
Poor performance particularly following bacterial or viral invasion.
Joeschke (1984) reported depressed serum levels following such
invasions

Natural sources
Apples, Blackberries, Rose hips

Herb sources

Alfalfa	Dandelion
Comfrey	Red clover

B complex Choline

Choline is considered an essential nutrient for all species, but little else
is known.

Equine requirements:
Unknown
Manufactured by the animal, probably synthesized in the liver

Assists in:
The regulation of metabolic process
Growth factors
Formation of acetylcholine associated with the transmission of nerve
impulses
Fat metabolism aiding energy production

Main signs of deficiency:
Poor growth
Haemorrhage in kidneys
Inability to synthesize fat

Natural sources

Sugar beet	Whole oats
Wheat bran	Soybean

Herm Sources
Alfalfa

Vitamin D: D₃ (Cholecalciferol) animal; D₂ (Ergocalciferol) plant

Fat soluble. The 'sunshine' vitamin, so called because it can only be manufactured if the body is exposed to sufficient sunlight, the ultra-violet end of the spectrum being the pertinent factor. Unfortunately, many animals are denied sunlight because of modern husbandry techniques. Vitamin D has been shown to function as a hormone rather than as a pure vitamin.

Equine requirements:
Levels unknown
   It has been demonstrated that 11 to 45 minutes of daily sunshine prevent vitamin D deficiency manifesting in growing chicks.

Assists in:
Mineralization of bone by acting with calcium and phosphorus
Essential for all functions associated with calcium and phosphorus
   (e.g. muscle activity)
Concerned with the auto-immune activity of cells
Concerned with the recycling of calcium via the kidney

N.B.: The ratio of calcium to phosphorus is crucial when determining vitamin D requirements. A ratio of 1.2 calcium to 1.0 phosphorus seem to be the requirement of adult stock. If this ratio of 1.2:1.0 changes, becoming narrower or wider, the requirement for a vitamin D increase occurs.

Main signs of deficiency:
Weak porous bones
Enlargement (in young animals) of knee and hock joints
Abnormal hyaline cartilage
Spontaneous fractures
Delayed epiphyseal closure (epiphysitis)

Herb Sources
Alfalfa (sun cured)
Plants only contain very small amounts of vitamin D and the body has
   ineffective methods of absorbing the vitamin from plants,
   presumably because sufficient is produced within the body by
   exposure to sunlight.

Vitamin E (Tocopherol)
Fat soluble. Unlike other fat soluble vitamins it is stored for a short period of time in the body and then any extra is eliminated in the faeces.
   Tocopherol is Greek for 'ability to bear young'. Vitamin E's repu-

tation for helping fertility is well known. Selenium associates with vitamin E and increases its power. Manganese needs to be present in the body for vitamin E to be effective.

The oxidation of body cells is the partial cause of ageing. Vitamin E has been used to retard ageing. (Synthetic E will not prevent the oxidation of Vitamin A.)

The blood flow is improved by vitamin E and it causes blood vessels to dilate or expand. It is an inhibitor of improper blood coagulation, thus it helps prevent blood clots. It has been called nature's blood thinner. However, unlike chemical blood thinners it does not cause haemorrhage.

Equine requirements:
Probably 223 ug/1 mg body weight

Associated with:
Antioxidant
Cell respiration
Inhibits platelet clumping
May work with B_{12}
Assists in reactions of creatine phosphate and adenosine triphosphate

Main signs of deficiency:
Muscle degeneration
Possibly linked to 'tying up' syndrome

Herb sources

Alfalfa	Linseed
Comfrey	Sunflower
Dandelion	Rose hip

Vitamin H (Biotin, Coenzyme R)

Water soluble; member of the B complex family. It is found in small amounts in all living tissue. It can be synthesized by the intestinal bacteria. It is essential to the metabolism of carbohydrates, proteins, fat and unsaturated fatty acids

Assists in:
Metabolism of carbohydrates, protein, fats, especially unsaturated fatty acids
Normal growth
Maintains healthy skin, sebaceous glands, nerves, and bone marrow
Hoof growth

Main signs of deficiency:
Poor hoof growth
Fatigue
Poor appetite

Natural sources
Wheat germ, Rolled oats

Herb Sources

Alfalfa	Dandelion	Kelp
Blue cohosh	Eyebright	Licorice
Burdock	Fenugreek	Marshmallow
Capsicum	Ginger	Mullein
Cascara	Goldenseal	Papaya
Catnip	Hawthorn	Red clover
Chickweed	Hops	

Vitamin K (Phytomenadione)

Vitamin K is named after the Danish word for blood clotting, *koagulation*. It is important in the production of the clotting agent prothrombin and in the conversion of glucose to glycogen (the form of sugar stored in the body for use as fuel). Vitamin K is produced in the intestines.

Assists in:
Promotes proper blood clotting
Reduces haemorrhage

Natural sources

Alfalfa	Corn
Carrots	Wheat bran and germ

Herb Sources

Alfalfa	Papaya	Slippery elm
Gotu kola	Safflower	Yarrow

Vitamin P (Bioflavinoids)

Water soluble. Vitamin P is named after paprika, the spice from which it was first isolated. Actually a bioflavinoid complex consisting of rutin, hesperidin and citrin. Found in the pulp of fruits and vegetables.

Vitamin P aids the functions of vitamin C in keeping collagen (the connective tissue of cells) healthy. It also aids the action of the capillaries in allowing nutrients in and body wastes out. Bio-flavinoids are called the capillary permeability factor. It controls the size of the tiny holes in the capillaries, keeping them large enough to allow nutrients through, but too small for viruses (that may cause disease) or blood cells (that could lead to haemorrhaging) to pass.

Assists by:
Working synergistically with vitamin C
Strengthens capillary walls
Protects against arterial degeneration
Builds resistance to disease

Natural sources
Rose hips

Herb Sources

Burdock	Red clover	Slippery elm
Dandelion	Rose hips	Cayenne

Vitamin U
Many people do not recognize that this vitamin exists. Very little is known about vitamin U.

Natural sources
Grasses

Herb Sources
Alfalfa

PABA (Para-amino-benzoic Acid)
Water soluble. Part of the B complex family. It is actually a vitamin within a vitamin since it is one of the basic parts of folic acid. It helps with production of folic acid in the intestines. If conditions are right PABA can be synthesized in the intestines.

It aids in the metabolism of protein, and helps in the assimilation of pantothenic acid.

PABA is antagonistic to sulpha drugs. Sulpha drugs combine with the same things as PABA so the one that is in greater quantity crowds the other out. PABA can make sulpha drugs ineffective and sulpha drugs can cause a PABA deficiency as well as deficiencies of folic acid and pantothenic acid.

Natural sources
Bran, Wheat germ

Herb Sources

Alfalfa	Dandelion	Horsetail
Blue cohosh	Eyebright	Kelp
Burdock	Fenugreek	Licorice
Capsicum	Ginger	Marshmallow
Cascara	Goldenseal	Mullein
Catnip	Hawthorn	Papaya
Chickweed	Hops	Red clover

Minerals and Their Herb Sources

Minerals constitute a collection of ingredients required by the body for its basic life maintenance processes. They have a number of functions:

- As catalysts
- To activate vitamins
- To become structural components

All plants extract minerals from soil. Free ranging animal species will graze the palatable herbage and during the digestive process the body systems extract the required minerals from the broken down plant matter. Herbs have a high mineral content, adding yet another resource to their obvious dietary attributes.

Minerals tend to be incorporated within the animal's structural architecture. For example, calcium and phosphorus are major components of bone and without them it forms incorrectly, cannot repair efficiently and cannot maintain the required structural design. However too much of one mineral, or too little of another, can result in a deficiency or incorrect balance between the numerous ingredients necessary for the body to be able to utilize its calcium/phosphate intake which is just as hazardous as a lack of either calcium or phosphorus. Minerals are not manufactured by the body and must be replaced by dietary intake. If the intake is insufficient for the body's requirements, minerals which are already involved in a functional role will be withdrawn for redeployment in another capacity which is deemed by the body to be of greater importance. Certain energy processes (for example, muscle activity) require a constant calcium supply and an inadequacy may well occur during strenuous work. Should this situation arise and not be rectified, calcium will be removed from bone structures and recycled for use in muscle work with obvious and severe repercussions.

The situation gets more complex once it is realized that for every process of metabolic activity and interaction, a specific vitamin is also required. A shortage, no matter where, in the mineral/vitamin chain will result in functional inefficiency followed by deficiency disease.

Minerals are more complicated than vitamins because they cannot be used by the body in their natural form – they need to be *chelated*. The body must first dissolve the mineral substance and then bind it to a protein molecule. Only then will the blood stream accept the product. Minerals which are not chelated are excreted; and if a mineral is not accepted, the vitamins it should activate or work with will in their turn become unusable.

In all species, but particularly in the equine athlete, calcium and phosphorus need to be considered as one. They also need an intimate relationship with the sunshine vitamin (D) but unfortunately this is disregarded far too often. Have the purveyors of additives or feed distributors spoken to you of vitamin D when discussing your horse's requirements? If they have, I must apologize.

Calcium and phosphorus contribute the major part of the mineral content of bone. Both are required for efficient muscle activity, and they are also involved in nearly every metabolic function of the body. Vitamin D enhances the correct absorption, retention, mobilization and deposition of both minerals. Loss of bone density leading to spontaneous fractures has been described by many authors including Krook and Lowe as far back as 1964, and confirmed by Cunha in 1990.

Calcium is an alkaline present in chalk, limestone and marble. When fed as an additive it is found in the form of a compound limestone (calcium carbonate), calcium fluoride or calcium sulphate. Phosphorus is highly reactive, and unlike calcium, it does not occur freely in a simplistic natural form. It is found combined with oxygen as phosphate. Phosphorus is a major component of all cells both in animals and in plants.

Unfortunately the levels of both minerals are highly variable in all feed. There are many factors to consider: species, maturity, soil content, soil pH, the underground rock strata, climatic conditions, the seed and leaf content, the age of the feed and the harvesting methods all contribute to the concentration levels. One type of food may be high in phosphorus but low in calcium (for example bran), but this can be balanced by introducing a high calcium/low phosphorus ingredient. The turnip has a 2:1 calcium:phosphorus ratio, so those who fed the humble mangold were not so stupid after all.

Essential minerals

The equine requirement values suggested are taken from *Nutritional Requirements* as expressed in North America (1989). They should serve as a *guide* for *maintenance* only – they are not appropriate for high level activity requirements.

Calcium (Ca)
Alkaline earth metal

Equine requirements:
0.31–0.68% per kg of diet expressed as 100% dry matter.

- Aids in metabolism and is essential to the muscles
- Must have sufficient vitamin D
- Calcium loss is retarded by exercise
- Emotional stress can flush calcium out of the system at a high rate

Positive effects:
Nerve function–impulse transmission
Nerves stress
Strong bones and teeth
Works with magnesium for cardiovascular health
Helps regulate the heart beat
Helps proper blood clotting
Muscle contractions
Iron metabolism
Helps vitamin C functions

Signs of deficiency:
Poor growth
Fragile bones
Muscle cramps
Weak muscles

Natural sources
Green vegetables

Herb Sources

Alfalfa	Fennel	Parsley
Aloe	Garlic	Poke root
Black walnut	Ginger	Red clover
Capsicum	Ginseng	Red raspberry
Cascara	Goldenseal	Rose hips
Camomile	Kelp	Rosemary
Comfrey	Marshmallow	Sage
Dandelion	Papaya	Slippery elm
		White oak bark

Phosphorus (P)

Symbolized as a compound, e.g. phosphorus and oxygen PO_4^{3-}

Stored and utilized structurally in the bones and teeth, phosphorus is abundant in the body, being present in every cell. It is thought that phosphorus plays a role in all the chemical reactions of the body. The form of phosphorus present in the cells and body fluids is called ATP (adenosine triphosphate). ATP is a substance which controls the energy release of the body. Magnesium sparks energy and phosphorus controls it. Without magnesium the body would not have any energy and without phosphorus controlling the energy, it would burn itself out. Phosphorus is essential to nerve functions, especially those of nerve impulse. The brain is largely made up of fats that have been chemically combined with phosphorus.

Equine requirements
0.17–0.38% per kg of diet 100% dry basis

Positive Effects
Normal healthy bones, teeth and gums
Cell metabolism
Important to nerve function
Helps nerve impulse
Normal kidney function
Necessary for niacin (vitamin B_3 assimilation)
Proper sugar metabolism
Assimilation of proteins
Helps convert nutrients to energy

Natural sources
Whole grains

Herb Sources

Alfalfa	Dandelion	Poke root
Barberry	Garlic	Red raspberry
Black cohosh	Ginger	Rosemary
Black walnut	Goldenseal	Sage
Blue cohosh	Hawthorn	Slippery elm
Capsicum	Kelp	White oak bark
Catnip	Papaya	Wood betony
Comfrey	Parsley	

Sodium (Na), **Chlorine** (Cl), **Common salt** (NaCl)

An electrolyte. The value of common salt has probably been appreciated since prehistoric times and it has always been a valuable trade commodity. The harvesting of salt from the sea constituted an important industry in many offshore islands until the 1960s when land-excavated salt replaced pure sea salt to a great extent, despite the fact that the latter, with its sea-based nutrients, actually does improve taste!

Equine requirements:
0.50–1.00% per kg of diet 100% dry basis
Horses sweat more than any other species. They lose salt when
    sweating as the sweat contains 0.7% salt.
    Once again there is a complication: potassium (K) balances the salt levels and too much potassium results in a salt deficiency. Conversely too much salt will aggravate potassium levels.

Positive effects:
Regulation of the balance of body fluids
Assists in maintaining heart function
Assists in the transmission of nerve impulses
Sodium, together with potassium, regulates the acid-base balance

Natural sources:
Rock salt. Allow *free* access (it need *not* be mineralized)

Herb Sources
All herbs contain small amounts of salt but supplementation is needed for animals whose work causes excessive sweating. It is essential to understand that excess sodium chloride (salt) and potassium will *not*

be stored for future needs; it will be excreted. As the regulation of body fluids is of the *utmost importance* and is *continually* adjusted, a salt excess over and above the *immediate* requirements of the body will be just as detrimental as a deficiency. It is *vital* to *replace* the lost electrolytes before the fluid balance of the body is seriously disturbed and the animal becomes *dehydrated*, with all the dangerous consequences. (I once knew an old stud groom who used to scrape the horses' diluted sweat into a bucket as he washed them off. This was then offered to them as a drink – much cheaper than electrolytes, and recycling waste.)

Potassium (K)
An electrolyte. It is not found free in nature and, like phosphorus, is found in combined forms. Potassium is sometimes referred to as *potash*. Carbonate of potash is the result of burning organic material and placing the residue in pots to allow it to cool and dry.

Equine requirements:
0.40–1.00% per kg of diet 100% dry basis
Works with sodium to balance the body fluids, to keep the acid/alkaline balance of those fluids and to regulate the heart beat. Potassium is necessary to move substances (nutrients, wastes, etc.) through the cell walls. The body uses what has been called a sodium potassium pump. Potassium works inside the cell walls and sodium works just outside the cell walls. Potassium and sodium are called electrolytes because they carry an electrical charge. It is this electrical charge that 'goes off' and allows the two electrolytes to pump the needed substances in and out of the cells. More potassium is needed by the body during any type of stress.

Positive effects:
Balances body fluids
Acid/alkaline balance of fluids
Helps transport oxygen to the brain
Helps convert glucose into glycogen
Balances sodium
Helps the body to grow normally

Natural sources
Carrots, Whole grains

Herb Sources

Alfalfa	Dandelion	Parsley
Aloe	Echinacea	Peppermint
Black walnut	Fennel	Raspberry
Blue cohosh	Garlic	Rose hips
Capsicum	Ginger	Slippery elm
Cascara	Goldenseal	Valerian
Camomile	Kelp	White oak
Chaparral	Mullein	Yarrow
Comfrey	Papaya	

Magnesium (Mg)
Alkaline earth metal. Found in compound forms – magnesite, dolomite, etc. It is necessary for metabolism of calcium, vitamin C, phosphorus, sodium and potassium. Vitamin B_6 helps in the utilization of magnesium. It is used by the body to spark energy (*see* also *Phosphorus*). Magnesium is lost in urine and faeces.

Equine requirements:
0.08–0.13% per kg of diet 100% dry basis

Positive effects:
Helps nerve functions
Helps muscle functions
Assists blood bearing of oxygen and carbon dioxide
Necessary for strong teeth
Sparks energy release in body
Helps bone growth
Prevents calcium deposits
Helps mineral metabolism
Helps acid/alkaline balance
Aids carbohydrate metabolism
Helps turn blood sugar to energy.

N.B.: The soil content of magnesium is decreased following heavy dressing with nitrogen and/or potassium.

Natural sources
Fresh green vegetables, Wheat germ.

Herb Sources

Alfalfa	Comfrey	Mullein
Aloe	Dandelion	Papaya
Black walnut	Garlic	Parsley
Blue cohosh	Ginger	Peppermint
Capsicum	Gotu Kola	Red clover
Catnip	Hops	Rosemary
Camomile	Kelp	Valerian
		Wood Betony

Sulphur (S)

Organic sulphur is necessary for all basic body metabolisms. It works with the B complex vitamins and is contained in vitamin B_1 (*thiamine*), vitamin B_5 (*pantothenic acid*) and vitamin H (*biotin*). Haemoglobin contains sulphur. Sulphur is found in all body proteins; in fact, it is considered a key ingredient in protein, aiding it in all its functions. It is lost in urine.

Equine requirements:
0.15% per kg of diet 100% dry basis

Positive effects:
Helps in production of collagen, building of tissue, body repair and maintenance
Helps antibody production
Helps fight bacterial infections
Aids liver in bile secretion
The liver has many enzymes containing sulphur
Aids carbohydrate metabolism
Attaches with pollutants so they can be removed
Incorporated in polypeptide chains
Aids carrying of oxygen in blood
Helps to maintain oxygen balance necessary for proper brain functions
Contained in insulin, adrenalin, and thyroxin

Natural sources
Wheat germ

Herb Sources

Alfalfa	Capsicum	Chaparral
Burdock	Catnip	Comfrey

Dandelion	Juniper	Parsley
Echinacea	Kelp	Peppermint
Fennel	Lobelia	Sarsaparilla
Garlic	Mullein	Thyme
		White oak bark

N.B.: Sulphur requirements are very low. Flowers of sulphur powder fed to horses can be poisonous (toxic).

Iron (Fe)
The necessity for iron, like salt, has been recognized since time immemorial. Iron is a component of every living organism. It is absorbed throughout the gastrointestinal tract (see the section on *Digestive system* in Chapter 1). The amount absorbed has been shown to be dependent not only on the source but also upon:

● The health of the animal
● Its age
● The balance of the partnership minerals required by iron to function usefully
● The state of the animal's intestinal tract
● Efficient function within the intestinal tract, in particular its pH state

Iron is lost in faeces, urine and heavy sweating after exertion.

Equine requirements:
40–50 mg/kg in diet, expressed as 100% dry matter

Positive effects:
Oxygen transport
Activation of oxygen
Functional activities of all cells
Binds to proteins for complex metabolic functions
Assists in immunity
Assists in auto-immune activity
Is involved in *all* body activities

Natural sources
Whole grain cereals, Oatmeal

Herb Sources

Alfalfa	Ginger	Peppermint
Aloe	Ginseng	Poke root
Burdock	Goldenseal	Red clover
Capsicum	Hawthorn	Red raspberry
Camomile	Hops	Rose hips
Chickweed	Horsetail	Rosemary
Comfrey	Kelp	Sarsaparilla
Dandelion	Lobelia	Skullcap
Echinacea	Marshmallow	Slippery elm
Eyebright	Mullein	Tahebo
Fenugreek	Papaya	White oak bark
Garlic	Parsley	Yarrow
		Yellow dock

Copper (Cu), Molybdenum (Mo)
Copper and molybdenum interact. Their joint role is not clearly understood, particularly that of molybdenum, but they perform important biochemical as well as nutritional functions.

Equine requirements:
10 mg/kg of diet 100% dry basis

Positive effects:
Plays an important role in immunity
Are involved in central nervous system functions
Assist and are essential for iron activity
Assist in collagen metabolism
Involved in health of coat
Involved in fat metabolism

Natural sources
Whole grains, Leafy green vegetables

Herb Sources

Burdock	Garlic	Peppermint
Chickweed	Goldenseal	Red clover
Comfrey	Horsetail	Sarsaparilla
Dandelion	Juniper	Slippery elm
Echinacea	Kelp	Valerian
Eyebright	Lobelia	Yarrow

Iodine (I)
Almost all of the trace mineral iodine goes to the thyroid gland to manufacture thyroxin. Thyroxin is a hormone which affects growth and metabolism.

Equine requirements:
0.10 mg/kg of diet 100% dry matter
Large areas of the planet are *iodine deficient.*

Positive effects:
The only known effects are associated with the thyroid – certain of the metabolic process.
Normal growth

Sources
Mineral rich drinking water
Herbage uptake is entirely dependent upon soil conditions
Fertilization with seaweed has been shown to improve herbage content

Zinc (Zn)
Throughout the ancient world zinc is reported as being used as an ointment to cure skin conditions. As with iodine, there appear to be large areas on the planet which are zinc deficient. Copper needs zinc and zinc needs copper for any process within the body. It is lost in sweat and faeces.

Equine requirements:
40mg/kg of diet 100% dry basis

Positive effects:
Bound to other elements, zinc assists in:
Immunity
Wound healing
Growth
Behavioural patterns
Genetic translation and transcription
Microbial growth
Fat metabolism
Protection of cell membranes
Water balance acting with sodium pumps

Natural sources
Wheat germ, Bran, Green leafy vegetables

Herb Sources

Aloe	Eyebright	Licorice
Burdock	Garlic	Marshmallow
Camomile	Goldenseal	Rosemary
Chickweed	Hawthorn	Sarsaparilla
Comfrey	Hops	Slippery elm
Dandelion	Kelp	

Manganese (MA)

Manganese is a trace material which is needed for normal bone growth and structure. It is a catalyst for vitamins B and C. It helps with the proper use of vitamin E. It is important to reproduction because it aids in the manufacture of sex hormones and lactation. Manganese also helps in the formation of thyroxin and in vitamin and carbohydrate metabolism.

Equine requirements:
40mg/kg of diet 100% dry matter

Positive effects:
Skeletal growth
Muscle reflexes and co-ordination
Important for normal central nervous system
Helps eliminate fatigue

Natural sources
Green leafy vegetables, Whole grains

Herb Sources

Aloe	Chickweed	Licorice
Barberry	Garlic	Red clover
Black walnut	Goldenseal	Red raspberry
Cascara	Hops	Sarsaparilla
Catnip	Horsetail	Wood betony
Camomile	Kelp	Yarrow
		Yellow dock

Selenium (Se)

The need for and feeding of selenium is a serious problem. Deficiency causes severe muscle disease. For example foals who have been carried by a mare with a selenium deficiency can hardly stand at birth. Older horses have presented with bilateral wastage of specific muscle groups: triceps, quadriceps femoris and the masseter (jaw) muscles. The heart muscle is also affected. *Excess* selenium is toxic (poisonous) to the extent that death can result.

Interestingly certain sources of protein, notably *linseed*, achieve a protection against the toxicity of selenium.

Once again the search for a sensible feed regime leads us back in time. At one time a *linseed mash* once, or sometimes twice a week, was a part of a stable routine. The 'feeders' had no scientific backing for their actions but obviously they had a reason and it can only have been improved equine health and performance.

Equine requirements:
0.10mg/k (max) diet, *only* if hay is deficient

Positive effects:
Helps clean cell membranes
Works with vitamin E

Natural Sources
Bran

Herb Sources

Garlic	Lobelia	Slippery elm
Kelp	Red clover	

Fluorine (F)
A highly toxic mineral which appears to be essential in most species. It came to prominence in 1979 when Mandel reported a reduction in dental caries in children if the water supply contained fluoride. Contamination by industrial pollution can seriously raise the amount of fluorine in herbage to toxic levels.

Horses affected by excess fluorine exhibit a dry rough coat, tight skin, excessive tooth wear, poor mastication and chronic pain in all four feet.

Equine requirements:
Levels required unknown.

In conclusion

As with vitamins, it is possible that the full complement of the planet's minerals are as yet undiscovered. The following *must* be present in minute quantities for health but are known to be toxic if consumed in any quantity over a long period:

Aluminium (Al)	Lead (Pb)
Arsenic (As)	Mercury (Hg)
Cadmium (Cd)	

Boron (B), lithium (Li), silicon (Si), and vanadium (V) come under the heading of 'newly discovered' trace elements. To a large extent their role is not fully understood but a total lack of any or all results in deficiency conditions.

It is difficult to portray the complexity of the interaction of every requirement of the living body. Visualize an orchestra and think of the pages of the score, covered with (to the non-musical) endless hieroglyphics. Each means something to every member of the orchestra, but some pages mean more than others to different musicians as the notes on those pages represent their special function as particular players. However without their instruments those players cannot fulfil their functions and each member of the orchestra must play his or her own role in order to produce a perfect rendering of the piece, be it the *1812 Overture* or Handel's *Messiah*. The orchestra is directed by the conductor who has the power to influence his players. Each conductor has his own individual interpretation of the score.

The challenges created by differing circumstances 'conduct' the way the body must respond – each system is a player, each player needs a complex instrument (think of the number of keys in a piano) with which he or she responds to those demands and all the players must harmonize for the final result – sometimes this will be perfect and sometimes not.

All that has been suggested in the previous pages are the benefits of allowing natural selection from fresh organic sources. Table 2.1 lists 13 common herbs in order to demonstrate the micronutrients (vitamins) and minerals which are available provided the plants were grown in soil not exhausted by intensive agriculture. It is *not* a complete list.

All the information is intended to promote health. It is for *nutritive* herbal use, not *curative* herbal use. Those who wish to 'treat' ill health or injury must seek veterinary advice as *no treatment* will be effective unless the *correct diagnosis* is first procured. Once a diagnosis has been made, a study of the medicinal properties of herbs is necessary for it is unwise to 'doctor' at random. In 1984 Juliette de Bairgeli Levy wrote the *Herbal Handbook for Farm and Stable* in which she quotes Louis

Table 2.1 Some common herb sources of vitamins and minerals.

	Alfalfa	Camomile	Comfrey	Chickweed	Dandelion	Fernugreek	Garlic	Hawthorn	Red clover	Rosemary	Raspberry	Sage	Thyme
Vitamins													
A	✓	✓	✓		✓	✓	✓		✓		✓	✓	
B$_1$	✓			✓	✓	✓	✓	✓	✓				
B$_2$	✓			✓	✓		✓		✓				
B$_3$	✓			✓			✓		✓	✓			
B$_5$*	✓			✓				✓					
B$_6$	✓			✓	✓				✓				
B$_9$	✓			✓	✓				✓				
B$_{12}$	✓			✓	✓	✓			✓				
C	✓		✓	✓	✓		✓		✓				✓
D**	✓	✓		✓		✓				✓			
E	✓	✓		✓							✓		
Minerals													
Calcium	✓		✓			✓		✓	✓	✓	✓		
Cobalt						✓			✓				
Copper			✓	✓		✓		✓	✓				
Fluorine	✓												
Iodine													
Iron	✓		✓	✓	✓	✓	✓	✓	✓	✓	✓		
Magnesium	✓	✓	✓		✓			✓		✓	✓		
Manganese		✓		✓				✓		✓		✓	
Phosphorus	✓		✓			✓	✓	✓		✓		✓	
Potassium	✓	✓	✓		✓						✓		
Selenium							✓		✓				
Sodium	✓			✓	✓			✓		✓		✓	✓
Sulphur	✓					✓	✓						✓
Zinc		✓	✓	✓	✓		✓				✓		

*   Manufactured in body
** Requires natural sunlight

Bromfield who in his book *Pleasant Valley* writes that any person in charge of land or animals 'has to know more things than a person in any other profession; he or she has to be a biologist, a veterinary, a mechanic, a botanist, a horticulturist, a stockman and many other things', certainly pertinent for the maintenance of health.

Of the various herbal sources listed as being 'producers' of the necessary vitamins and minerals it must be obvious that alfalfa (lucerne) is a very nutritious plant. The plant originated in Asia and was taken by merchants to Greece and from there began Roman usage. 'The Romans were well acquainted with its properties as a forage plant, particularly for horses' wrote Henry Stephens, FRSE in 1851.

The plant is described in most comprehensive herbals, particularly those of European origin. *Modern Practical Farriery* published in 1881 and *The Book of the Farm* published in 1851 both devote large sections to alfalfa. The crop is said to increase yield annually, reaching maturity in three years. Both authors stress the necessity for a good dressing of 'old yard manure'. Sprangle in 1775 in his paper *The Improved Culture of Lucerne (Alfalfa)* describes 81 species – I wonder how many are available today?

When discussing hay, the publications mentioned stressed that 'upland meadow' 8 months old was best. Much emphasis is placed on the time of cutting, the number of 'forage' plants required, the time allowed for wilting and the care which must be exercised to avoid excessive seed or leaf loss.

I rather fear modern methods do not allow for such considerations and this is unfortunately a problem difficult to overcome if you are trying to feed a yard full of horses. As a trainer said in despair, 'I simply cannot feed as my father and grandfather did – I cannot get the stuff they used'.

For the single horse owner a 'patch' of alfalfa is quite easy to install, but remember to feed it well, preferably with seaweed.

Cycles of health

When considering athletic activity and the cycles for health it should be remembered that:

(1) Many of the components required by the body's factories are not stored for future demand. The body has no ability to plan for the future, and therefore no reason to store surplus for an unpredictable possible demand.

(2) The components required for extra or excessive activity can be increased (i.e. storage levels raised) in response to increased exercise demands, so while there is a fine line between too much and too little, if the demands are a *constant* the body will adapt its process of manufacture to meet them. But it will expect a constant balanced demand level, thus if you are training for a 3 mile

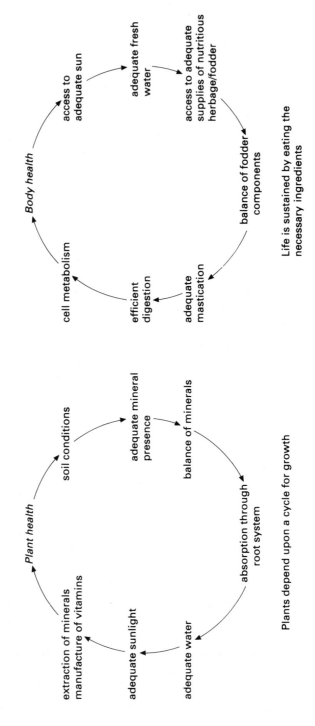

Fig. 2.1 Cycles of health.

gallop with the horse expected to carry 12 stone, its ability to perform adequately for the '3 miles, 12 stone' demand is unrealistic if it has only been carrying 8 lbs and walking 5 miles a day!

(3) The availability of replacement components for those used during activity is an essential post-activity requirement for adequate recovery. If there is no access to the essential components the body will borrow/extract from its own tissues the materials required for repair/restoration/replenishment following exertion. This will 'weaken' and render less efficient the structures from which components have been 'borrowed'.

Supplements

Supplementation is poorly understood, and there is a dearth of *proven* experimental information on the absolute levels of minerals required for horses. Maintenance levels are *suggested* but even the requirements of human athletes are constantly adjusted with the discovery of 'new' minerals and vitamins. One thing is certain – the amounts required are remarkably small and oversupplementation is toxic. Free choice supplementation is the best approach. Supplementation really should not be necessary if the quality of herbage contains adequate minerals/vitamins to start with.

I once attended a lecture on feeding for endurance competitions. The lecturer described his paddocks, the way he made hay and the oats and maize he grew. His horses were only fed his own forage, they looked magnificent, the pastures were old untouched meadows and he proudly pointed out they contained 74 species! He was kind enough to send me a list (see Table 2.2). Subsequently I discovered he was on a green sand belt. Lucky owner, lucky horses.

The storage of forage, no matter what type, is *very* important. Most minerals and vitamins are unstable and adversely affected by changes in temperature, humidity, packaging, compression or an over-dry atmosphere. The 'new' types of Haylage try to prevent loss by packaging in a vacuum but the minute the seal of the vacuum pack is broken the contents begin to oxidize and therefore change. Be careful how and where you store. If the container says 'reseal', reseal, and if there is a 'use by' date the product will be of no benefit and may even do harm if used after that date. Put yourself in your horse's place – you don't eat outdated produce so why should your horse?

A note of caution: herbs affect body metabolism. They can interact

Table 2.2   The 74 species found in an old meadow. (There is no record of the meadow ever having been ploughed.)

Scientific name	Common name	Scientific name	Common name
Arrhenatherum elatius	False oat-grass	*Prunella vulgaris*	Selfheal
Poa pratensis	Smooth meadow grass	*Cirsium vulgare*	Spear thistle
Festuca ovina	Sheep's fescue	*Plantago media*	Hoary plantain
Helianthemum nummularium	Common rock-rose	*Centaurea nigra*	Black knapweed
Filipendula vulgaris	Dropwort	*Carex flacca*	Carnation sedge
Plantago lanceolata	Ribwort plantain	*Thymus praecox*	Wild thyme
Dactylis glomerata	Cock's-foot	*Achillea millifolium*	Yarrow
Pimpinella saxifraga	Burnet saxifrage	*Carduus nutans*	Musk thistle
Urtica dioica	Common nettle	*Briza media*	Quaking grass
Medicago lapolina	Black medick	*Reseda lutea*	Wild mignonette
Galium verum	Lady's bedstraw	*Ranunculus repens*	Creeping buttercup
Trisetum flavescens	Golden oat grass	*Silene vulgaris*	Bladder campion
Phleum pratense	Timothy grass	*Myosotis arvensis*	Field forget-me-not
Holcus lanatus	Yorkshire fog	*Potentilla reptans*	Creeping cinquefoil
Crepis capillaris	Smooth hawk's-beard	*Galium mollugo*	Hedge bedstraw
Campanula glomerata	Clustered bellflower	*Vicia cracca*	Tufted vetch
Bromus erectus	Upright broom	*Fragaria vesca*	Wild strawberry
Trifolium pratense	Red clover	*Brachypodium pinnatum*	Tor grass
Campanula rotundifolia	Harebell	*Plantago major*	Great plantain
Agrostis stolonifera	Creeping bent-grass	*Pastinaca sativa*	Wild parsnip
Centaurea scabiosa	Greater knapweed	*Anacamptis pyramidalis*	Pyramidal orchid
Sanguisorba minor	Salad burnet	*Succisa pratensis*	Devil's-bit scabious
Primula veris	Cowslip	*Scabiosa columbaria*	Greater knapweed
Tragopogon pratensis	Goat's-beard	*Polygala calcarea*	Chalk milkwort
Taraxacum officinale	Dandelion	*Gentianella amarella*	Autumn gentian
Cirsium acaulon	Dwarf thistle	*Asperula cynanchia*	Squinancywort
Veronica chamaedrys	Germander speedwell	*Picris hieracioides*	Bristly ox-tongue
Arenaria serpyllifolia	Thyme-leaved sandwort	*Stachys officinalis*	Betony
Cerastium fontanum	Common mouse-ear	*Rumex acetosa*	Common sorrel
Senecio vulgaris	Groundsel	*Sambucus nigra*	Elder
Sonchus asper	Pricky sow-thistle	*Koeleria macrantha*	Crested hair-grass
Linum catharticum	Fairy flax	*Ligustrum vulgare*	Wild privet
Leontodon hispidus	Rough hawkbit	*Rhamnus catharticum*	Alder buckthorn
Lotus corniculatus	Common bird's-foot trefoil	*Betula pendula*	Silver birch
Senecio jacobaea	Common ragwort	*Trifolium repens*	White clover
Leucanthemum vulgare	Ox-eye daisy	*Viola hirta*	Hairy violet
Knautia arvensis	Field scabious	*Crataegus monogyna*	Hawthorn

adversely with chemicals i.e. orthodox drugs if chemical medication is being administered. *They may also increase threshold levels of body substances which 'enhance performance' above those established as normal.* The prohibited substance list is very extensive and lays down parameters for what are known as *prohibited substance levels*. These are established and refer to any agents that influence:

- The central nervous system
- The autonomic nervous system
- The cardiovascular system
- The gastro-intestinal function
- The immune system and its response

They act as:

- Antibiotics
- Antihistamines
- Anti-malarials and anti-parasitic agents
- Anti-pyretics, analgesic and anti-inflammatory substances
- Diuretics
- Local anaesthetics
- Muscle relaxants
- Respiratory stimulants

They influence:

- Sex hormones
- Endocrine secretions
- Substances affecting blood coagulation
- Cytotoxic substances

It is important to realise that 'going alternative' rather than 'using orthodox' does *not* mean your horse will automatically *'test negative'*. However provided your horse has been allowed a 'balanced' intake rather than an 'excess' all will be well. This knowledge leads us to the practice of another 'green' approach: *homoeopathy*.

Useful addresses

National Institute of Medical Herbalists
9 Palace Gate
Exeter
Devon EX1 1JA
Tel: 0392 426022

School of Phytotherapy (Herbal Medicine)
Bucksteep Manor
Bodle Street Green
Hailsham
East Sussex BN27 4RJ
Tel: 0323 833812
Fax: 0323 833869

Further reading

de Bairgeli Levy, J. (1984) *Herbal Handbook for Farm and Stable.* Faber & Faber Ltd, London.

Lust, J. (1990) *The Herb Book.* Bantam Books, London.

McDowell Lee, R. (1989) *Vitamins in Animal Nutrition.* Academic Press, London.

McDowell Lee, R. (1992) *Minerals in Animal and Human Nutrition.* Academic Press, London.

Mervyn, L. (1984) *The Dictionary of Vitamins.* Thorsens Publishers Ltd, London.

Mervyn, L. (1985) *The Dictionary of Minerals.* Thorsens Publishers Ltd, London.

Mollison, B. (1991) *Introduction to Permaculture.* Tageri Publications, Australia.

Stuart, M. (1987) *The Encyclopedia of Herbs and Herbalism.* Macdonald and Co, London.

Vogel, H.C.A. (1990) *The Nature Doctor.* Mainstream Publishing Co (Edinburgh) Ltd, Edinburgh.

Part II
Therapies

3   Homoeopathy

Introduction

There is some confusion about the differences between herbal medicine and homoeopathic medicine, particularly as both derive their basic ingredients from natural resources. The main difference can be understood when it is appreciated that in homoeopathy there is no standard remedy for a known condition. Each individual case should be separately assessed and a specific remedy prescribed. The remedies will vary and those chosen should be related to the whole. This must take into account the environment, personality and character as well as the symptoms experienced. Current medical thinking is that it is the symptoms of a condition which need to be treated; homoeopathy considers that the symptoms are the reactive efforts or responses of the body's defence systems to an invasion and these symptoms need to be stimulated rather than suppressed. The principal of *similia similibus curentur* (let like be treated by like) is employed in order to achieve this.

Hippocrates, the fifth century BC Greek physician, recognized this, as did the Swiss alchemist, Paracelsus, in the sixteenth century but it was left to Dr Samuel Hahnemann, born in Saxony in 1755, to 'rediscover' the idea. It was he who evolved the name *homoeopathy* from the Greek language – 'homois' for like and 'pathos' for suffering. Hahnemann was obviously remarkably gifted, he spoke nine languages, he was a chemist and then became a Doctor of Medicine, and it was while translating the *Materia Medica* of Professor Cullen of Edinburgh that he began to experiment upon himself. When he took quinine (or as it was then known Cinchona bark), a known remedy for malaria, he found that he developed symptoms indistinguishable from those of malaria itself. A little later, in 1796, Dr Edward Jenner used the secretions from cows with cowpox to vaccinate people and prevent them from contracting smallpox.

Hahnemann continued to experiment by giving single remedies to volunteers. Between 1779 and 1832 his research contributed 112 papers. Substantial proof was required by the apothocaries of the day whose medical practices included bleeding, cupping and the use of toxic elements such as arsenic, repeatedly prescribed in ever larger quantities if a cure was not effected. Proof of Hahnemann's ability to cure by his methods came in 1821 when the battle of Leipzig ended with a typhoid epidemic. Hahnemann treated 180 cases and only one patient died. In 1831 of the 154 cases of cholera he treated, only 6 died, while of the 1500 treated by the then 'orthodox' methods 821 died. The principles handed down from Hahnemann form the basis of the practising homoeopaths of today.

Arguments continue as to the validity of homoeopathic remedies, due in the main to the dilution of the initial component. Hahnemann dosed his healthy volunteers with various substances and continued until they produced symptoms resembling a known illness. Once it was established that a particular substance had evoked a symptom or symptoms it was subjected to *dynamization*, with one drop of the *mother tincture* (substance) being diluted with 99 drops of alcohol and the mixture shaken vigorously. This shaking (*succussion*) is essential for the preparation of remedies and the process is repeated until the required dilution (*potency*) is achieved. Hahnemann had 'proved' 99 mother tinctures before his death in 1843.

Today the preparation of homoeopathic remedies still uses the processes of dynamization and succussion to achieve the required potency, exactly as described by Hahnemann, despite the fact that it has been scientifically proven that after the ninth dynamization not a single molecule of the original substance remains. Critics claim the effects are placebo. If this is so, why do homoeopathic remedies prove so beneficial in animal therapy?

Questions and theories abound: Can such an infinitesimal dose permeate the cell membrane? Can disorientated receptors recognize the energy imprint of the original and use it to restabilize? Does the remedy set up vibratory interactions disturbed by toxic reactions? Whatever the reason, homoeopathy undoubtedly has a role both in prevention and cure.

As with any extrinsic interference, it is unwise just to buy a remedy and 'try it'. Homoeopathy evolved after much experimentation by a medical man who was also a chemist. He understood, even though limited by eighteenth century knowledge, the problems of health and the signs and symptoms of disease. The science he recognized is practised successfully by people who have been trained at specialist schools, many of whom have previously qualified as doctors or vets.

Homoeopathy requires considerably more observation than orthodox medicine so you can help your homoeopathic vet by constant surveillance. You should note down the behaviour of your horse and its reactions over a period of time. Listed below are some of the factors to which your horse may react and which will help your homoeopathic vet in his general assessment:

Climate:
Heat, cold, humidity, rain, thunder, wind, sun.

Diet:
Barley, oats, bran, nuts, mixes, linseed, sugarbeet, horseage, meadow hay, lucerne hay, water.
Drinks a lot, drinks little, eats up, leaves food, eats earth, licks a lot of salt.

Bedding:
Paper, shavings, straw.
Eats bedding, digs.

Temperament:
Restless, temper flashes, over-sensitive, dull.

Reaction to rider or groom:
Angry, friendly, moves away, no co-operation.

Posture:
Leans, sits on walls, always lying down, never lies down, rolls constantly, rests a leg, points a leg.

Sensations:
Sweats easily, in patches, for no reason. Itches, paws the ground, crib bites, wind sucks, legs swell (hind only swell, front only swell), resents girth or roller, cold backed.

Pain:
Disunited, avoids a lead, will not bend on a circle, rests a leg, head shakes, avoids contact with the bit, kicks out for no reason, bucks for no reason, rolls often, bites sides, looks tucked up.

General health:
Speed of healing, spotty coat, dull coat, dehydration, sparse thick

urine. Eats droppings, dry droppings, sloppy droppings, bad
breath, quids food, runny nose, runny eyes, pale gums.

Never well since:
Medication, cough, accident, colic, vaccination, anaesthetic, competition, fall race, change of diet, change of bedding.

General appearance:
Alert, dull, dry coat, pale gums, pale round eyes, poor hoof growth,
cats hairs under jaw remain despite coat change, runny eyes, early
fatigue, slow cardiovascular recovery after exhaustion.

First aid

If you, the owner, or groom have a good relationship with your
homoeopathic vet it is helpful to have a small selection of remedies for
first aid. These can be purchased either from the vet or a good
homoeopathic pharmacy, such as Ainsworths in London. The
potencies of homoeopathic remedies are indicated by a number. This
may be followed by the latter x. For example 6x potency contains
$\frac{1}{1\,000\,000}$ part of the total original substance. Those remedies styled
'high' potencies (200th, 1r, 10r, etc.) are those with the most minute
amounts of the basic preparation. The most commonly used potency
on sale to the general public is 6x, and most qualified practitioners
dispense from their own pharmacies.

Suggested first aid kit
In the absence of professional advice choose the remedy most
appropriate for the situation. *Do not* give the animal several remedies
in case one is 'better' than another.

Aconite (*Aconitum napellus*) Common monkshood
Uses: Relieves pain, sedates temporarily.
Of the same family as the buttercup, the plant grows in damp areas in
south west England and south Wales.
The remedy is obtained from a part of the root system.
The plant is poisonous to carnivores but less so to herbivores.
The remedy can be in tablet or liquid format.

Arnica (*Arnica montana*)
Uses: Bruising both superficial and deep. Filling in joints.

The plant grows in the mountain pastures of central Europe where the soil is calcareous.

The remedy is obtained from the flowers and rhizomes.

The remedy can be in the form of tablets, lotion or cream.

Belladonna (*Atrope bella-donna*) **Deadly Nightshade**

Uses: Pain killer, tissue antispasmodic, anti-asthmatic, all via its effect on the nervous system.

The plant grows throughout southern England. It is poisonous, particularly to species with a highly developed nervous system. It should never be used if bleeding is occurring as its effects are to increase rather than decrease haemorrhage.

The remedy is obtained from the leaves and roots.

The remedy can be taken as a tablet or used as a tincture.

Hypericum (*Hypericum perforatum*) **St Johns Wort**

Uses: Grazes, broken skin, bruised nerves.

The plant grows throughout the UK in dry sunny positions.

The remedy is obtained from the tips of the fresh flowers.

The remedy can be taken in a fluid or as a syrup. A fluid extract or oil can be applied directly to the damaged area.

Witch Hazel *(Hamamelis virginiana)*

Uses: Reduces bleeding by constricting blood vessels. Useful for immediate first aid for tendon strain.

The plant grows as a garden shrub in the UK and it is found in the wild state in North America.

The remedy is obtained from the leaves.

The remedy is best applied as a tincture or infusion externally over the damaged area.

With experience, the basic first aid kit will obviously grow and contain an increased number of remedies. As so many seem to have similar effects, the burning question is: 'how do I decide which to use?' You must ask yourself questions. Aconite and belladonna both relieve pain, but do you need general sedation as well as pain reduction or do you need to ease pain and reduce tension in the tissues after local damage? Aconite relieves pain but also sedates. Belladonna reduces pain and relieves local spasm. If the horse has had an accident and is upset aconite might be the choice but if the horse has been kicked belladonna would possibly suit better. You must try to choose the remedy most appropriate to the symptoms and the individual's needs.

Many of the plants sources used in homoeopathy to aid the body to recover from adverse occurrences are classified as poisonous, that is they are toxic in their natural state. Once the remedy has been extracted and been subjected to the processes associated with achieving the correct potency, and provided the prescribed dose is *not* exceeded, the effects of the substance will be to neutralize the adverse effects of the condition for which it has been shown to be pertinent.

Homoeopathy, like herbalism, is effective. It is classified as 'alternative' but this does not mean it is easy to use. In fact it is far more difficult than pursuing orthodox medical methods, *but* patients who turn to homoeopathic medicine find they are healthier and the reports from owners using homoeopathic vets give similar results. It must be understood that it is not a DIY substitute. *The general attitude that alternative therapies are 'easier' and can be prescribed and practised by anyone could not be further from the truth.* Alternative therapies present a greater challenge, there are no fixed formulae, no fixed rules and the goal posts are continuously on the move.

Bach Flower Remedies

No account of homoeopathy would be complete without a mention of the Bach Flower Remedies. Dr Bach was a doctor of medicine who first worked in public health, then studied bacteriology. In the early 1900s, dissatisfied with orthodox medical attitudes he turned to homoeopathy as he, like Hahnemann, was certain that the emotional state of the patient contributed to their health problems.

His training as a bacteriologist led him to examine the intestinal flora of patients in his care. Intestinal flora are bacteria normally present within the intestines, even in health. Bach discovered that chronic conditions changed the normal patterns of these flora and each condition gives rise to its own peculiar archetype of disturbance. Bach isolated seven groups of intestinal flora and from nosodes, using homoeopathic principals, he prepared remedies. A nosode describes material extracted from the product of a disease. The patient is 'dosed' with a minute amount of the product in order to effect a cure.

The use of a preparation extracted from the saliva of dogs with rabies had been used to cure humans suffering from hydrophobia as early as 1833, so the practice was not new. However the main difference was that after he isolated what are still called the seven bowel (intestinal) nosodes Bach prescribed the appropriate remedy not after considering the patient's symptoms (for example, the fever, colic, a cough, pain) but according to the emotional state or temperament of the person. A patient suffering from a stomach ulcer would be treated for worry/anxiety, the remedy used being chosen as appropriate for that patient's mental condition. Orthodox medical practitioners were not convinced despite, at this stage in his career, the scientific background to the work.

In 1930 Bach left London and moved to the country to seek remedies from nature for emotional states. It is said he became highly mentally and physically sensitive. In a self-described 'negative' state of mind he would set off and wander through unspoilt country until he chanced upon a flower which he felt restored his mental and physical serenity. Between 1930 and 1936, when he died, he had chosen 38 flowers from trees and plants to counteract what he considered were the 38 adverse mental states which man might experience, disease-induced or not. The remedies could, he considered, be used to prevent the onset of physical conditions as the mental state was relieved.

Despite the fact that all the work relates to human disease and the intestinal flora of the human gut, the Bach Flower Remedies are used by many people for their animals. Animals are undoubtedly temperamental but it is the owner who will interpret and classify their horse's 'mood'. This leads to the distinct possibility of an incorrect assessment and consequently the use of an inappropriate remedy.

Many people carry Rescue Remedy which is a conglomerate of five of the 38. Described as a remedy for emergencies it is evolved from:

- Clematis to avoid fainting
- Cherry plum to control hysteria
- Impatiens to relax physical and emotional tension
- Rock rose to avoid fear and/or panic reactions
- Star of Bethlehem to alleviate shock

For the average horse the suggested dosage would be ten drops in the water bucket or four drops on a sugar lump.

The *mother tinctures* of all the remedies are prepared using the petal tips of the fresh flowers from the appropriate plants. Just as with other complementary therapies, correct selection is the most important factor for success. The art of prescribing requires an in-depth study of equine mentality and its response to stress. Very little published work is available. If the remedies are as effective as they are claimed to be, misreading a situation would make things worse rather than better.

Useful addresses

The Faculty of Homoeopathy
2 Powis Place
Great Ormond Street
London WC1N 3HJ
Tel: 071 837-2495

The British Homoeopathic Association
27a Devonshire Street
London W1N 3BR
Tel: 071 935-2163

Further reading

Blackie, M.G. (1984) *The Challenge of Homoeopathy*. Unwin Paperbacks, London.
Chiej, R. (1984) *The Macdonald Encyclopedia of Medicinal Plants*. Macdonald and Co, London.
Livingston, R. (1991) *Homoeopathy, Evergreen Medicine*. Asher Press.
Macleod, G. (1983) *The Treatment of Horses by Homoeopathy*. Eastern Press Ltd.
Macleod, G. (1983) *A Veterinary Materia Medica*. The C.W. Daniel Co Ltd, Saffron Walden, Essex.

4 Acupuncture and Acupressure

Acupuncture

For acupuncture to be successful, no matter which technique is used to influence the *points*, it is essential to understand that by triggering even just one reaction, because of the interaction of all the systems of the body, any influence by one system upon another will concern and affect the whole.

In the west we tend to think of acupuncture as a single therapy. This is an incorrect concept as acupuncture is a part of the 'whole' in traditional Chinese medicine, just as surgery is a part of the whole of western medicine. Just as you cannot practise surgery without a diagnosis and a knowledge of anatomy and disease, no-one should practise acupuncture unless they understand the basic principles of the philosophy of Chinese traditional medicine.

It was not until the early 1970s that acupuncture began to be extensively practised in the west, despite the fact that Chinese records date back to 2697 BC. Possibly this apparent lack of interest stemmed from the fact that the philosophy behind Chinese medicine which requires the whole, not just the symptoms to be considered, was alien to western medical practice, wherein the symptoms were treated and the whole rarely considered. Chinese medicine aims to achieve *balance* and prevent sickness; western medicine treats the after-effects of sickness and passes the search for the reason to 'another department' with the patient getting little or no advice to enable them to help themselves. This, coupled with long medical names and incomprehensible information, often leads to problems which are exacerbated by fear. The Chinese approach embraces already accepted and therefore 'fearfree' concepts. The facts that balance is necessary (not only throughout the body but also in life) and the terminology is not alien but relates to the components of daily living (light, fire, water, sweat, bitter, spicy) means people already have experience of such things and can relate similar characteristics in matters of health or illness, be it their own or that of their animals.

Basic principals of traditional Chinese veterinary medicine

Yin and yang

Early teaching considered that there were principal underlying laws which governed the universe, both metaphysical and physical. These theories, which became laws, stated that there was a constant interaction between opposites as those opposites endeavoured to achieve balance. These phenomena are known as *yin* and *yang*.

Yin is considered to have a negative or passive quality and yang is considered to have active or positive qualities. Every organic and inorganic object within the known universe was classified as being either yin or yang. The organs, their functions and reactions are classified as *ts'ang* (yin or passive) or *fu* (yang or positive). Each organ is considered to need to interact with all the other organs, and for good function to be achieved there must be balance throughout the whole. The Chinese consider an upset of the yin to yang balance creates a situation which allows for the onset of disease or for a state of being unwell.

Unfortunately acupuncture cannot correct imbalance by directly influencing yin or yang – it rebalances by manipulating *ch'i* or energy. It is considered that the body contains *meridians* which are described as paths interlinking all the body organs, not only to each other, but also to the body surface. The *ch'i* (which may be yin or yang) flows in a specific pattern within this network. The specific points for acupuncture are located on the *paths* of meridians.

Influencing a *point* will affect energy flow and this flow in its turn will affect the organ associated with the point. Not only will the functions of that organ be activated, but the effects of its functions will influence and create activity within all the other organs which specifically react with the one first stimulated. Depending on the *ch'i* required (it may be yin or yang) and the type of organ, which in turn may be a *ts'ang* organ (relatively solid: heart, lung, liver, spleen and kidney) or a *fu* organ (hollow: gall bladder, small intestine, stomach, large intestine and bladder) so the effects required are executed via a point stimulation and a very complex chain reaction.

Because of the multiplicity of interaction between the meridians, the body organs and energy, the stimulation of one point may not be effective and, if needed, other harmonizing, enhancing points will be selected.

The range of points is immensely complex and choice must relate not only to the need for balance but also the interdependence of the whole, both within itself and within the environment.

The five elements

Wood, fire, earth, metal and water are considered to be the primary materials from which the universe is composed. These five are not static. They are all continually passing through the processes of growth and metamorphosis. Their interactions create and destroy, and involve the transformation of both living and non-living materials. The life of animals and humans also complete five changes which correspond to natural changes. The interlinking is shown in Table 4.1.

The philosophy of the five elements is difficult to explain in a literal western manner for there are no equivalent or comparable thought processes in western attitudes. The *creation* within the five elements is conceived thus: *wood* burns and creates *fire*; the resulting ash becomes *earth*, which contains minerals and *metal* is made from minerals. In a moist atmosphere condensation on metal forms *water* and the water feeds vegetation thus completing the cycle by recreating *wood*.

Destruction limits overproduction as the roots of the tree (*wood*), stretching into the earth, absorb nutrients thus destroying *earth*. Water flow is limited by a dam made of earth, thus earth destroys *water*. *Fire* destroys *metal* by melting it and metal shaped into tools destroys *wood*.

The fundamental rule is equilibrium. If any process dominates, be it creative or destructive, balance is lost. The striving to maintain balance is of paramount importance. Even though acupuncture is conceived primarily as a means of maintaining health, 'diagnosis' is required to ensure the organs are functioning normally and any deviation, however small, should be corrected before a yin/yang imbalance has resulted in malfunction or, as it is termed in the west, disease.

Diagnosis

Even in a healthy animal a decision regarding the points to be stimulated can only be arrived at after a step-by-step analysis of the animal's physical appearance as well as its demeanour. *Observation* is

Table 4.1 Traditional Chinese analysis of nature and living beings.

Categories of fives

Elements	Wood	Fire	Earth	Metal	Water
Stages of life	Embryo	Adolescence	Adulthood	Old Age	Death
Seasons	Spring	Summer	Late summer	Autumn	Winter
Directions	East	South	Centre	West	North
Ch'i	Wind	Fire, heat	Moisture	Dryness	Cold
Tsang organs	Liver	Heart	Spleen	Lung	Kidney
Fu organs	Gallbladder	Small intestine	Stomach	Large intestine	Urinary bladder
T'i	Muscle	Blood vessels	Fat	Skin and hair	Bone
Ch'ao orifices	Eye	Tongue	Mouth	Nose	Ear
Fluids	Tear	Sweat	Saliva	Mucus	Urine
Pulses	Taut (hsien)	Full (huang)	Slow (ch'ih)	Light (fu)	Deep (ch'em)
Colours	Green	Red	Yellow	White	Black
Tastes	Sour	Bitter	Sweet	Spicy	Salty
Functional processes	Germination	Growth	Maturation	Fruit production	Dormancy

of paramount importance in Chinese veterinary medicine. As every horse adopts a differing stance, be it at rest, standing, lying or while at work, the normal of that animal needs to be recognized before an accurate diagnosis is possible.

The four steps required for *diagnosis* are

(1) *Observation:*
  (a) Lips: changes in lip colour are considered to indicate problems in the spleen and as the spleen and stomach are closely linked, lip changes also implicate the stomach.
  (b) Urine: bladder problems.
  (c) Droppings: stomach and intestines.
  (d) Limbs: hoof problems.
  (e) Skin: spots or pustules indicate blood and *ch'i* abnormalities.
  (f) Tongue: heart involvement.
(2) *Listening:*
  (a) Breathing sounds: rasping, dry, stiff sounds all indicate lung disorders.
  (b) Grinding of teeth or crib biting are associated with kidney disorder.
  (c) Intestinal rumblings: Chinese veterinarians have classified each sound and related it to a specific area of the intestines.
(3) *Questioning:*
  The owner is asked about appetite, respiration, droppings, urination, and the smell of breath, urine and droppings. The owner's observations are then related to the sex, age, size, breed and workload of the animal.
(4) *Palpation:*
  (a) General body palpation will indicate tender areas. These areas are noted for each will correspond to a specific organ. Surface temperature and sensory responses are evaluated.
  (b) Pulse readings are taken from six sites on the front of the chest just lateral to the trachea (windpipe) – three on the right (the *three gates*) and three on the left (the *three portions*). The gates (*feng, ch'i* and *ming*) are associated with various organs, as are the *upper, middle* and *lower* portions.

  Gate associations are
  - *Feng:* lungs and large intestine.
  - *Ch'i:* spleen and stomach.
  - *Ming: Ch'i* of the kidney and the triple burner (heater).

Portion associations are:
- *Upper:* heart and small intestine.
- *Middle:* liver and gall bladder.
- *Lower:* kidney and bladder.

Each pulse is taken three times and each time the pressure is increased.

- *Fu:* lighter superficial pressure.
- *Chung:* medium pressure.
- *Ch'en:* very deep pressure.

Each of the readings is described by its quality:

- *Ping mo:* a normal regular pulse, which in the horse at rest is 36–44 beats per minute.
- *Fan mo*, a reverse pulse, abnormal in any one of several ways:
  Fu mo – very 'light'.
  Ch'en mo – requires deep pressure to locate it.
  Ch'ih mo – slower than normal.
  Shu mo – rapid.
  Hsien mo – feels like a taut string.
  Huang mo – forceful.
  Hua mo – almost fibrillating, one beat 'rolls' into the next.
  Sse mo – intermittent, weak.
  K'ou mo – has a hollow feel.
  Hsi mo – feeble beat.
  Each of these reverse pulse findings indicate to the trained practitioner a state within the animal's systems. The location at which the pulse variation was noted will give some indication of the organ involved. Thus if the pulse taken at the *ming* gate is found to be *hsien mo*, a kidney problem of obstruction involving both *ch'i* and circulation could be present. The correct points on the appropriate meridian need to be stimulated to adjust and balance the kidney and its associates before irreversible changes happen or disease manifests.
  The pulses are considered so important that a further five *yie mo* (changed pulses) need to be appreciated. These pulses changes are *very* subtle and require great sensitivity

of touch to appreciate the minute but very important variations.

● *Yie mo* or changed pulses are as follows:

A *picking pulse* – irregular rhythm with a missing beat after every third or fourth beat. Associated with a toxic condition.

A *leaking pulse* – feeble beats with an irregular rhythm. Associated with the heart.

An *entangled pulse* – feels very superficial and is intermittent. Associated with a toxic condition.

A *dashing pulse* – superficial feel, irregular and is felt as a rush then pause. Associated with gastro-intestinal problems.

A *puffing pulse* is reminiscent of the bubbles rising to the surface as water boils. Associated with failure within the five *tsang* organs (see Table 4.1).

Pulse appreciation is considered important for both diagnosis and prognosis.

The triple burner or triple heater

The triple burner (see Fig. 4.1) is collated to the five *fu* organs (see Table 4.1). It has no single fixed anatomical location; nor is it entirely responsible for any specific organ. It is considered to influence functions, i.e. blood flow, lymphatic flow, *ch'i* movement, digestion, secretion and absorption. It is the transport and exchange stimulator. It is called *triple* as it is considered in three distinct sections: the upper, middle and lower burners each influence an area rather than an organ.

Upper burner: facilitates body defence and lung function.
The area is forward of the diaphragm and therefore embraces the front third of the horse. Included in this area are the lungs, heart, cranial thorax, neck and the head.

Middle burner: facilitates digestion and nutrient delivery.
The area lies behind the diaphragm and ends at the level of the umbilicus. The spleen, stomach and cranial abdominal contents are within this region.

Lower burner: functions to maintain fluid drainage.
The final third of the horse, from umbilicus to tail, contains the liver,

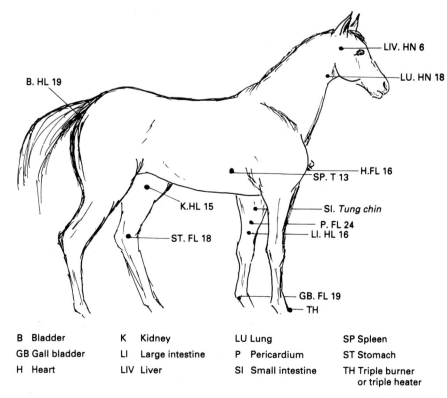

B. HL 19

LIV. HN 6

LU. HN 18

H.FL 16

SP. T 13

K.HL 15

SI. *Tung chin*

P. FL 24

LI. HL 16

ST. FL 18

GB. FL 19

TH

B	Bladder	K	Kidney	LU Lung	SP Spleen
GB	Gall bladder	LI	Large intestine	P Pericardium	ST Stomach
H	Heart	LIV	Liver	SI Small intestine	TH Triple burner or triple heater

Fig. 4.1 The twelve (traditional) meridian points. For accuracy each point must be located with reference to the Chinese text.

large and small intestines, kidneys, bladder and organs of reproduction.

The appropriate sections of the triple burner require stimulation when diagnosis has identified malfunction in any of the functions it appears to influence.

Meridians (connecting energy paths)

The meridian network is not as comprehensive for animals as it is for the human subjects. The work of the traditional Chinese acupuncturists describes 12 meridian points (see Fig. 4.1). *Remember*, the organs have their own stimulation points; the meridians are concerned purely with energy (*ch'i*) flow.

Modern western charts have extended the meridians relating to the horse and this has caused considerable controversy. In Oriental countries the points and meridian points described and used were compiled in 1972 at the Lanchau Veterinary Research Institute. These points and charts relate to the 1608 work *Yuen Heng Liao Ma Chi*. Veterinarians in Europe and America have transposed human meridians onto animal charts.

The rapid increase in the use of acupuncture as an alternative therapy has unfortunately led to confusion in application. There are many reasons for this: Romanizing Chinese characters is not straightforward as there are several methods, each with a differing system, as many Romanizers failed to appreciate the subtle nuances of the various dialects. As many charts bear little or no relationship to their originals it is small wonder acupuncture is less successful in the west. Undoubtedly those practitioners who have remained faithful to traditional Chinese points achieve the best results. For those readers who wish to practise medical acupuncture on their horses, a knowledge of the body functions, the ability to recognize both beneficial and adverse effects, a precise anatomical appreciation and a diagnosis preferably made by a qualified veterinary surgeon are essential, particularly when considering the fact that many of the cases seen in the twentieth century had no equal in 1608. Thankfully, conditions such as gangrene, tetanus and convulsions have, to all intents and purposes, disappeared. However laminitis, lung disorders, tendonitis still occur in the twentieth century horse, but you should not expect to find viral disorders described.

Point stimulation

Traditionally very fine needles are inserted beneath the skin at selected points. The penetration depth varies depending on the locality of the point. Successful needle insertion gives rise to a definite response – as the needle sinks in the operator will feel a tightening around it. It feels 'steady' and will remain in situ without support. A loose needle that apparently falls about has missed the point. Once the needle is correctly sited the acupuncturist will rotate it both clockwise and anticlockwise until an increased tissue resistance is felt as the needle becomes tightly grasped. Needles of various lengths and gauges are sold in sets.

In the UK the Veterinary Act prohibits the insertion of needles into any animal by anyone other than a qualified veterinary surgeon.

However, the low level laser can be used to stimulate points and finger pressure is equally effective. Learning to work with the fingers has the advantage of improving the tactile sensitivity of both the operator's fingertips and thumbs (an essential for successful massage) and as this sensitivity increases an appreciation of minute temperature changes and variations in tissue tension can also be recognized, all of which are helpful when using palpation to aid diagnosis.

Laser acupuncture

Those who use low level lasers in a random fashion to 'treat' areas of the horse which they consider to be painful (for example, the back) are quite unwittingly stimulating acupuncture points. Several low level lasers have multi-diode heads. The surface area of the applicator may be 1 to $1\frac{1}{2}$ inches in diameter and to 'treat' a horse's back with such a laser and miss the acupuncture points would require considerable skill. Passing a laser with a multi-diode head down both sides of a horse's back from withers to dock could influence as many as 38 points. In view of the elaborate procedure undertaken by a veterinary acupuncturist *before* treating a horse in order to make certain that the points selected will complement each other and achieve balance and harmony, the activation of a mass of contradictory, rather than complementary, points is irresponsible.

Great care must be exercised with any form of therapy. Although low level lasers *are* able to stimulate superficial acupuncture joints, some doubt has been expressed about their efficacy for deep sited points. Muscle damage, muscle pain and muscle stiffness can all be helped using low level laser acupuncture, *but* unless the actual site of the pain is discovered, the origin and site of the cause identified, the appropriate points stimulated and the *ch'i* of the appropriate meridian enhanced, the problem will not resolve.

In order to address a condition in a responsible manner, the lack of precision of the multi-diode head makes it inappropriate when an exact location is necessary for effective therapy. In this instance the greater accuracy of the single diode laser should be employed.

Acupressure (Traditional Chinese Methods)

For *puncture* substitute *pressure*. Pressure techniques (*shiatsu*) are practised by the Japanese, and the Chinese who term the method of stimulation *tui nor*. The *acu* points are stimulated either by using small metal balls, a ball being placed over the point deemed to require stimulation, or by finger pressure. The balls are pushed down and inward with the palm of the hand, or left in situ on the surface, held in place by adhesive tape. This method has found favour for the treatment of travel sickness when the metal balls are securely mounted on elastic bands and sufferers invited to place the bands around their wrists with the ball on the centre of the underside of the wrist. The *pericardium* channel of *hand-jueyin*, which originates in the chest, is mapped anatomically from the chest to the front of the armpit (*axilla*), then down the upper arm adjacent to two other channels, the lung channel of *hand-toiyin* and the heart channel of *hand shauyin*, to the front of the elbow where it crosses the depression (the *cubital fossa*). Continuing downward centrally on the front of the forearm, it reaches the wrist and lies between the tendons of two forearm muscles (the *palmaris longus* and the *flexor carpi radialis*). There are two points (the *neiguan* and the *daling*) at the wrist, both of which control gastric pain, vomiting and panic (see Fig. 4.2).

Small spherical magnets mounted on bands are currently popular for pain relief. It would be nearly impossible to attach effectively either a small metal ball or small magnet to a horse, particularly as the skin of a horse is considerably more mobile than that of the human. As will be seen in the description of point sites, points are located via skin resistance but if the skin moves, the underlying point will be lost.

The ball of the thumb is most useful for applying pressure to points, although some people prefer a fingertip or, for huge muscle masses such as the muscle of the quarters, the point of the elbow can be used.

Effective acupressure needs exactly the same approach as acupuncture.

First of all *diagnosis* should take place, leading to a consideration of:

- The selection of the appropriate points (5 to 15 are usually needed)
- The selection of the appropriate meridian
- The consideration of yin to yang
- The *ch'i* requirements

Point location

The area of the skin above all the various acu points exhibits considerably less resistance to the passage of weak electrical currents than

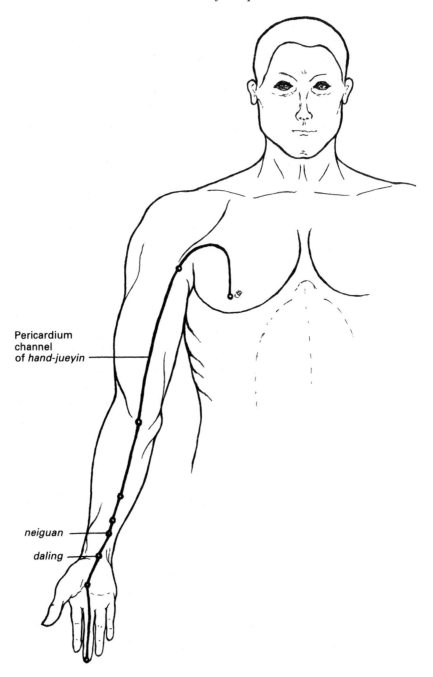

Fig. 4.2 Points which in a human can control gastric pain, vomiting and panic.

does the surrounding skin. This lowered resistance can be detected by skilled operators who describe the point areas as having a slightly differing texture, being in small depressions, or feeling softer. It is impossible to practice *acu*, be it puncture or pressure, without a chart depicting and numbering the points, the textbook relevant to the chart and an anatomy book. The relevant text to chart is essential as each school of acu describes in a manner dependent on the original translation.

All points are described anatomically for example, 'between the processes of T11 and T12', 'in the depression between the spinous processes of C1 and C2', 'in the fossa beside the junction of the scapular cartilage and the anterior angle of the scapular', hence the need for an anatomy book, particularly one which includes surface anatomy. The distance from anatomical landmarks has also been carefully calculated: *tsun* is a measurement of length. The width of the 16th rib, at the point where an imaginary line from the *tuber coxae* (point of hip) crosses that rib, is considered in each individual to be one *tsun*. (Each *tsun* is divided into ten *fen*.) To calculate the *tsun* a pair of dividers is placed accurately over the 16th rib at the appropriate site which will give an accurate width that can be measured. The *tsun* calculated is appropriate for that individual only. In the point location chart the anatomical description will not only describe the anatomical landmarks but may also include *2 tsun* from point *x*, and in the needling/pressure charts *2–3 fen deep* will denote a superficial point, while *3–5 fen* denotes a deep point and needle or pressure must be applied accordingly.

Because of the differing skin resistance point finders have been developed. In effect these are searching electrodes. The tip of the 'finder/detector' is sensitized to record the minute variations within the skin's surface. When an area of lowered resistance is encountered the apparatus will emit a bleep or a light (usually red) illuminates. This all seems very simple, so why waste time with *tsun* and anatomical landmarks? Unfortunately *any* skin change will be detected – a small patch of dried sweat, dirt in the coat, or dampness. Even searching an area with the detector, because it is electrical, will change the skin's resistance, as will local damage such as bruising, or temporary compression if the horse has been lying down, has had a tight roller or has been standing resting a leg. The very mobile skin of the horse is a further complication. Tests on dead animals show the lowered resistance is in the skin only, not in the underlying tissues, so a point 'found' by a point detector must always be double checked by using the anatomical landmarks and *tsun* measurements described in the text.

Point selection

Health maintenance rather than disease treatment is the purpose of this book, and carefully selected points can and do influence body function, even when an animal is apparently in good condition. The selection of points will depend upon what you wish to achieve: Was the horse stiff after work? Is the urine thick and strong smelling? Is the horse restless? All the steps described earlier under the heading *Diagnosis* in the section on Acupuncture need to be considered. Your decision must be carefully calculated, having determined the systems/organs/areas you wish to influence by a series of logical deductions after considering your horse as a whole. The points appropriate to the problem can then be selected by reference to the chosen chart and text. A London firm (Acumedic) stock a model horse with points marked and an accompanying text.

All basic texts describe around 114 points pertaining to the 'organs'. Each organ is governed by several points and each point will execute an effect fractionally different from other points which influence the same organ. No matter how small, that difference is critical when selecting a stimulation protocol. *Correct selection is the key to success or failure.*

Meridian selection

Traditional Chinese medicine describes 12 meridians (see Fig. 4.1 and Table 4.2) in the horse but only indicates one point for each meridian. This is unusual as meridians are normally multi-point endowed. Westernization has extracted points from human meridian charts and allocated them to the horse, and in doing so the number of points has extended from 12 to 350!

Once the organ has been selected its governing meridian will need stimulation and its yin or yang requirements must be balanced by the release or containment of *ch'i* (remember, yin and yang cannot be influenced directly to regain their necessary equilibrium – this is achieved through ch'i).

Table 4.2 The 12 traditional meridians. A yin always has an opposite balancing yang.

Yin meridians have *t'sang* organs	Function	Yang meridians have *fu* organs	Function
Liver	Resistance to disease Stores nutrients Influences blood transport	Gall bladder	Hormone balance Nutrient distribution
Heart	Blood control Transportation Helps body to respond to external stimuli	Small intestine	Digestion Food adaptation
Spleen	Aids digestion	Stomach	Classifies and regulates food intake

Lung	Extracts and
	    manipulates *ch'i*
	Excretes toxic gas
		Large intestine	Separates substances,
			    both solids and
			    liquids, to be
			    excreted

Kidney	Controls fluids	Bladder	Excretes polluted fluids

Pericardium	Protects heart *ch'i* in
	    disease
		Triple heater	Circulates energy
			Influences all transport
			    and exchange

N.B.: The functions listed are taken from traditional Chinese thinking. They are merely indications of functional organ influence. The concepts *do not* relate directly to western observations, but they have lasted successfully for several thousand years.

Application of pressure

Suggested pressure requirements for different points are:

Superficial points	2–3 *fen*	5 lb or less
Medium-sited points	1–2 *tsun*	10–15 lb
Deep-sited points	2–5 *tsun*	15 lb

The only way to learn your own strength is to experiment with a set of calibrated weighing scales. Using the finger or thumb, you intend to work with, push on the scales until you register the various weights suggested. You must then mentally note the sensation of thrust and transpose it to the pressure points.

While no type of point stimulation should cause the subject discomfort, occasionally resentment is apparent during stimulation or on the following day the horse may seem to be less comfortable than it was prior to therapy. Reappraisal is necessary in such situations. The techniques are supposed to be beneficial and while the benefits may not be immediately apparent adverse results indicate an incorrect diagnosis and or point selection.

Technique for acupressure

- The horse should be relaxed standing on a non-slip floor in stocks or in his own box.
- The operator should run their hands over the horse to accustom the animal to their touch and pressure. This is called *opening*.
- The points must be identified accurately by feel or detector.

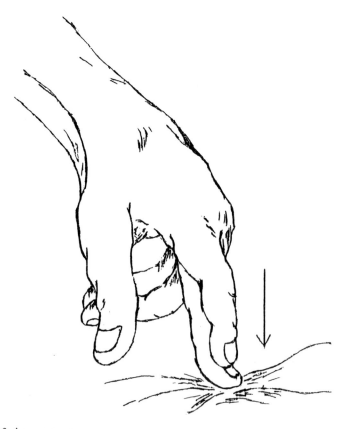

Fig. 4.3 Acupressure.

- Pressure is applied with thumb, fingers or elbow placed not at an angle but perpendicular to the point. Stimulation calls for pressure application at the approximate poundage necessary for each individual point. The pressure should be applied using a small circular movement. The time required for each condition will vary and should be indicated in your chosen text.
- Work the points from the head toward the tail and/or from the top toward the ground.
- After all the points have been stimulated on one side move to the other, but *remember* some points are single as they are centrally situated.
- On completion of the second side, again run the hands over the horse as a final relaxation or *closing*.

The number of sessions required will depend on the results. Once a week is quite adequate as a 'top up' to maintain health. Over-stimulation wastes body resources. Remember the minute amounts needed in homoeopathic remedies.

Chen points

Figure 4.4 shows the traditional Chinese acupressure points from the *Chen Needle Classic* chart.

D before the number indicates a deep point and S a superficial point. TH is the triple burner (see also Fig. 4.1).

Points to stimulate for fatigue (Chinese), stress (western) and the triple burner

S2	Bilateral:	Three *fen* from the medial field of the nostrils on an imaginary line running from the lower border of one nostril to the other.
S9	Bilateral:	Two *tsun* from the top of the nostril rim at its upper part.
S10	Bilaterial:	One *tsun* from the top of the nostril rim at its upper part.
D47	Single point:	In the depression between the spine of the first sacral spine and last lumbar spine.
S59	Single point:	The tip of the last tail vertebrae (tip of dock).

Pulling the ears gently will also relieve stress. Ear points are marked on

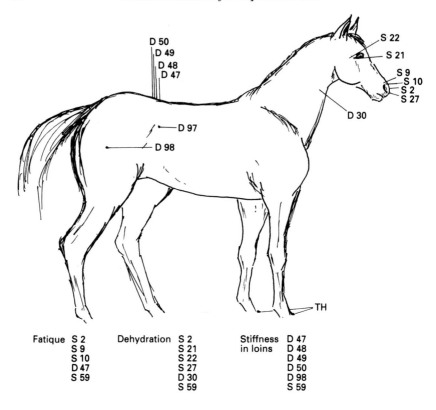

Fatique	S 2	Dehydration	S 2	Stiffness	D 47
	S 9		S 21	in loins	D 48
	S 10		S 22		D 49
	D 47		S 27		D 50
	S 59		D 30		D 98
			S 59		S 59

Fig. 4.4 Chen points.

many early charts but are not documented in the book, *Veterinary Acupuncture*. Ginioux, working in France, considers several points beneficial and I use several with success in stressed animals (see Fig. 4.5). Westmayer considers one useful (see also Fig. 4.5).

Points to stimulate for sunstroke (Chinese), dehydration (western) and the bladder meridian

(See Fig. 4.1 for the bladder meridian.)

S2 Bilateral: Three *fen* from the medial field of the nostrils on an imaginary line running from the lower border of one nostril to the other.

S21 Bilateral: On the transverse facial vein, 1 *tsun* behind and below the outer edge of the meeting of the eyelids.

S22 Bilateral: Five *fen* behind point 21.

S27 Bilateral: On an imaginary line between the lower border of the nostril 3 *fen* in.

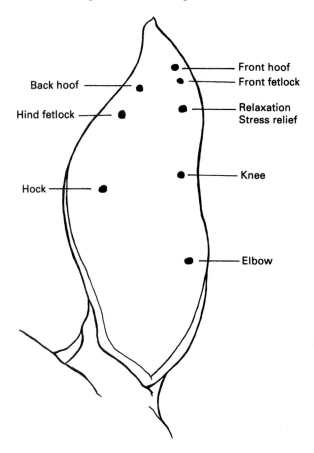

Front hoof
Front fetlock
Back hoof
Relaxation
Stress relief
Hind fetlock
Knee
Hock
Elbow

Fig. 4.5 Ear points after Ginioux and Westmayer.

D30 Bilateral: Mentally divide the jugular vein into three sections, the point is at the junction of the upper and middle one third.

S59 Single point: The tip of the last tail vertebrae (tip of dock).

Points to stimulate for muscle stiffness in the loins
(Find 50 first.)

D47 Bilateral: Two *tsun* in front of 48.
D48 Bilateral: Two *tsun* in front of 49.
D49 Bilateral: Two *tsun* in front of 50.
D50 Single point: In the depression between the spine of the first sacral spine and the last lumbar spine.

D97 Bilateral: On an imaginary line stretching from the dorsal midline to the tuber coxae point located on the lateral third of the line.

D98 Bilateral: Midway between the convexity of the trochanter of the femur and the patella.

S59 Single point: The tip of the last tail vertebrae (tip of dock).

These are just three very basic prescriptions using the traditional approach. Although traditional methods have often been significantly altered to accommodate western ideals, it does not mean they will not be effective. It may be that they are less effective than the original versions but the science has been adapted for twentieth century conditions. All science develops from basic concepts and all students need to appreciate the ground rules of any subject. Those who wish to pursue acupressure or acupuncture should, if they have grasped this section of text, have no difficulty in expanding their interests in either the traditional or the western styles. However, there are no short cuts in any of the complementary, as opposed to orthodox, therapies; all demand an in depth appreciation of factors involved. Massage can and does complement acupressure, but it is also a subject on its own.

Further reading

All the titles listed here are available from Acumedic, 101–103 Campen High Street, London NW1 7NJ.

Essentials of Chinese Acupuncture, (1980) compiled at Beijing College, Foreign Language Press, Beijing.

Ginoux, D. (1986) *Soulagez Votre Cheval aux Doigts*, Pierre-Marcel Foure, 2 rue du Sabot, Paris.

Klide, Alen M. & Kung, Shiu 4. (1986) *Veterinary Acupuncture*, 3rd edn. University of Pennsylvania Press, USA.

Koptchuk, Ted J. (1983) *The Web That Has No Weaver*. Rider and Co, London.

Westermayer, Edwin (1979) *The Treatment of Horses by Acupuncture*. Health Science Press, Holsworthy.

Part III
Massage and Stretches

5 Muscles and Massage

Introduction

To the discerning reader it must be obvious that herbalism, homo-eopathy, acupuncture or acupressure requires in depth study in order to practise any one of the therapies safely and effectively. There is no instant learning curve and it is beyond the scope of this book to teach all the detail of the subjects. The aim is to expose readers to the complexities of age-old methods concerned with health. All the sub-jects were originally learnt in the traditional way by an apprentice-ship that lasted for years under a master. Massage is a less complicated subject and the section concerned with muscles aims to educate readers so they can practise effective massage on their own horses.

The Veterinary Act restricts the treatment of any animal to the owner, unless the vet in charge of the case authorizes treatment from a therapist. Thus persons who become proficient at massage and passive stretching *must* seek veterinary approval before working on animals other than their own.

Chapter 6: *Hand Preparation and General Points for the Masseur* suggests a safe professional approach for the would-be masseur, should he or she wish to work under veterinary supervision. The wearing of a kennel coat even when working on one's own animal not only protects clothes but is useful because the horse will soon learn that massage is pleasurable and will associate the pleasure with a familiar routine – horses are far more observant than they are given credit for.

Go slowly as a beginner – Rome was *not* built in a day. I hope you will derive as much pleasure in learning to use your hands, as your horse will benefit from your efforts.

Muscle structure and function

In order to massage usefully it is important to understand the structure of muscle, its work, capabilities, training response, acquired problems, work efforts, nerve control, feeding, cleansing, regenerative properties and response to toxins, as well as the types of muscle and the differing roles required to enable your horse to respond to your demands as a rider, and for him to perform the complex movements the differing disciplines demand.

The body contains three distinct types of muscle tissue:

- Cardiac muscle
- Smooth muscle
- Skeletal muscle

Cardiac muscle.   The walls of the heart are composed of muscle. The heart must pump continuously from birth until death, it must be able to increase both the heart rate (speed) at which it pumps and, under the duress of strenuous exercise, it must increase the volume of blood it expels at each beat, thus it must increase its stroke volume.

In order to nourish its muscle the heart enjoys a blood supply (the coronary supply) independent of that of the main body. The heart also has a specialist nerve supply via the parasympathetic vagi and recurrent laryngeal nerves, and a control centre – the sino-atrial node (pacemaker).

Smooth muscle.   The cell structure of smooth muscle is suited to, and utilized for, constructing and forming the walls of some of the tube-like vessels, arteries, veins, as well as some of the organs, for example, the intestines.

Skeletal muscle.   For the purpose of this text *muscle* will refer to *skeletal muscle.* The properties of skeletal muscle allow for the conversion of chemical energy, delivered via the circulatory system, to mechanical energy. By utilizing the lever system of the bones of the skeleton, movement is achieved as muscles, using their contractile abilities, force one lever to act upon another.

Composition of skeletal muscle

Two types of protein (thin *actin* and stronger, thicker, *myosin*) bond their microscopic filaments together to form *myofibrils*. These in their turn are packed in thousands within a sheath to form the next architectural miracle – a muscle bundle. The bundles massed together form a working unit of muscle. Individual muscles have an internal fibre arrangement which will complement, in the most economic fashion, the functions demanded of them. Thus a *fusiform* arrangement is found when a large movement range is required and the *multipennate* arrangement features great power, but has a limited range (Fig. 5.1). The directional lie of the fibres is of great importance to the masseur.

Nerve supply to muscles

No muscle can function without a nerve supply. Commands from the central nervous system are delivered to the muscle's control centre (the motor end plate), via the motor nerve servicing the muscle. Chemical changes are initiated at the motor end plate in response to the commands from the central nervous system and the appropriate action results. In order to achieve coordinated movements, the changes which occur as muscles work must be recorded by sensory nerves and transmitted back to the central coordinating area within the brain.

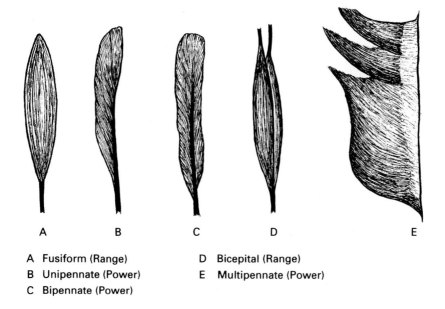

A	B	C	D	E

A Fusiform (Range)   D Bicepital (Range)
B Unipennate (Power)   E Multipennate (Power)
C Bipennate (Power)

Fig. 5.1 Muscle fibre arrangement.

Circulatory supply for muscles
Blood is responsible for the delivery of nutrients and removal of waste from muscles. An adequate supply of nutrients (including oxygen) is essential for muscle activity. Oxygen is required continuously by some muscle fibres, but only for waste removal by others. The rapid removal of the waste products generated by activity is of paramount importance because of its potential toxic qualities.

Large arterial vessels divide and subdivide within the muscle structure impregnating the tissue with a plexus of vessels. These continue to divide until each individual muscle cell is eventually supplied with capillaries. The capillaries deliver the food and take in the waste which is moved to venules, then on to the veins and slowly carried, via the venous system, to the excretory vessels. Excess fluids not accepted by the veins are absorbed by lymphatic vessels lying adjacent to parts of the venous system. Massage assists in the removal of waste following activity.

Muscle fibre types
Three fibre types have been identified within the composition of skeletal muscle in the horse. They are classified by the difference in the speed of contraction and their need for oxygen. Differing breeds exhibit the three fibre types in differing proportions (Snow and Guy, 1980).

(1) *Slow twitch fibres* – ST (Slow oxative – SO)
   - These fibres contract slowly and relax slowly.
   - They are dependent upon oxygen for efficient function.
   - They are able to store fats as a source of energy.
   - They store relatively little glycogen.
   - They have a reddish appearance as a result of their rich blood supply.
   - They are bulky.
   - They are stamina fibres.

(2) *Fast twitch fibres*
   (a) FT I (Fast glycolytic – FG)
   - Their contractile properties are rapid.
   - They can function in the absence of oxygen.
   - They have larger glycogen stores than do ST fibres.
   - The circulatory network is not as dense so the removal of waste is less efficient.

(b)   FT II (Fast oxative glycolytic – FOG)

● These fibres display some characteristics of both previous groups.
● They respond to exercise demands and build accordingly. Thus it is possible to either increase their capability to work in an anaerobic capacity increasing speed or build their endurance capabilities.

Conditioning muscle

Muscle responds and builds according to the demands placed upon it, but the ability to accept and cope with greater demands can only be achieved if certain criteria are met, or indeed if the animal has inherited the necessary muscle characteristics. Thus an animal mainly endowed with FT I fibres and who is conditioned to working at speed over short distances cannot be expected to suddenly work efficiently over a longer distance as its muscles do not have the capacity for such a sudden switch of effort. The muscles will need retraining to utilize any ST fibres they may have, but primarily to improve and build convertible FT II/FOG fibres.

● Muscle takes time to respond to a new training regime.
● To improve endurance the circulatory supply must be given time to build.
● The necessary energy sources must be available for conversion.
● The liver (a glycogen store) must have time to accommodate to the increased demands and improve its storage capacity.
● Heart and respiratory ability need to be improved.

The work of Snow & Guy suggests:

● Speed and power require a high percentage of FT I and FT II fibres (FG and FOG).
● Endurance requires a high percentage of ST (SO) fibres.

In the early stages of conditioning it is inadvisable to be in a hurry. If the animal is 'well covered' it is also necessary to decide if this is because it is fat or if its shape is due to muscle mass.

Conditioning requires regular and increasing activity. It cannot be achieved in one short daily exercise. Once fit a horse will only remain in that condition if exercise continues. One hour of activity a day is adequate for this. Muscles unused to new activities tire quickly. They need short bursts of activity followed by a short time to relax and recover, i.e. a pattern of work, relax; work, relax.

A horse's inability to perform a new task can be due to muscle fatigue, or lack of muscle power or a combination of the two. All muscles perform better if warmed up before they work and massage is of great benefit in this situation. Post activity muscle stiffness can also be reduced by massage.

Fatigue in muscles

Waste accumulation

Following exercise lactic acid forms in cells in the absence of oxygen. The complex metabolic processes associated with muscle activity give rise to many chemical changes and retention of the correct pH level is crucial. If the acidic levels change, so too do the metabolic processes; as they change they upset enzyme activity and eventually the incorrect chain reaction totally suppresses muscle contraction. Lactic acid is a by-product of activity. An excess of it acts as an irritant to muscle and causes stiffness and cramp. This type of cramp is *not* the cramp associated with 'Monday morning tying up' (see the section on *Rhabdomylosis*).

Excess lactic acid is removed from working muscle, as is other post-exercise debris, via the circulation. Normally it takes between three to four hours for muscle to be cleansed, *but* light exercise following strenuous exercise has demonstrated an ability for muscle to convert the waste lactic acid into an energy substrate provided oxygen is present. This enhances clearance, thus the lactate levels in the blood are reduced more rapidly if the animal is trotted for a period immediately following strenuous work. Respiration and heart rates must return to normal before a period of trotting commences to ensure there is no oxygen debt.

Glycogen depletion

The second reason for muscle fatigue is concerned with glycogen. Fatigue occurs rapidly when all the available glycogen has been used. Although fats can be used their rate of energy production is less efficient than glycogen and the muscles will slow their rate of contraction significantly. It takes approximately two days to replenish glycogen stores. Once again light exercise has proved to be beneficial in the two days following strenuous activity for, just as with lactic acid removal, light work appears to hasten the process of replenishment. Massage enhances both lactic acid removal and glycogen replacement processes by influencing circulatory flow.

Rhabdomylosis (tying up)

Tying up is a complex situation and studies have elicited differing clinical profiles with variable findings. However in all cases the muscle enzyme levels (CPK) are elevated, the gait is stilted, there is an acute pain response when affected muscle groups are palpated (most usually those over the loins), and the condition induces muscle damage. Unfortunately once affected, horses are likely to experience recurrent episodes.

Although tying up was considered originally to occur as a result of the high lactate levels created by exercise, a Swedish study has shown affected areas to be alkaline rather than acid with the possibility that calcium might be a culprit. Calcium is necessary to control many of the metabolic activities during muscle contraction. However as yet the pathophysiology of tying up has not been satisfactorily explained and prevention is also random – most owners and head lads have their own cures! Massage can help relax the muscle tension but must be carefully administered in such cases as the muscles do not respond normally.

Sprained or torn muscles

If muscle fibres break down under excessive strain, the torn fibres leak their chemical components and these chemicals act as a signal to the local circulation, resulting in an increased blood flow to the area. Swelling and pain (both a consequence of free chemicals) and increased local pressure occur, and the action of the affected section of the muscle is curtailed. Massage assists recovery.

Muscle function

As already stated, muscles use the bones as levers, but no lever can work without a fulcrum. Because of the complexity of the equine skeleton each muscle is required to fulfil a variety of specific, named roles.

Fixator: a muscle or group increase internal tension to create an immovable area in order for movement to occur elsewhere.

Primemover: a muscle or group which initiates a movement.

Antagonist: a muscle or group opposing the primemover but lengthening as the primemover shortens, in a manner which ensures a flowing movement within the segment. As the movement reverses so do the roles, with the antagonist becoming the primemover as the original primemover changes to play the role of antagonist.

The increased tension within a muscle may be:

Isometric: the working muscle or group function by increasing tension but not shortening.

Isotonic: the working muscle or group anticipate the function and contract slightly to achieve a state of readiness.

Concentric: this describes a muscle that is shortening as it works.

Eccentric: muscle activity describing a muscle that lengthens as it works.

Differing actions call for muscles to work within three ranges. Imagine a geometric protractor; the lever to be moved lies along the 180° base line and is broken at the 90° angle line.

Outer range: this is the most difficult as the muscle must work from 180° inward to about 145°. The lever is long and in its start position the muscle is at full stretch.

Middle range: the most effective and least tiring movement occurring from 145° through 90° to 45°. Muscle functions very efficiently in its middle range.

Inner range: the muscle works through a decreasing 45° angle. There is strength but little movement and this range causes fatigue.

Static work: Muscles only have to achieve a working tension and are unable to contract or relax. They fatigue rapidly.

Active work: a muscle working actively contracts and relaxes, the constant changes of tension within the muscle bulk ensuring adequate circulatory assistance, the result of the pumping actions around the vessels within the muscle.

While it would seem reasonable for active work to cause fatigue, in fact it is less fatiguing than static work.

Muscle work

It is important to study the biomechanics of the various equine sports in order to decide which muscle groups are likely to be the most fatigued. For example dressage with its demands for static, isometric work in the inner range for all the muscles of the neck is *very* exhausting.

Equine limbs are attached to the main body frame via ball and socket joints – the hip at the back and the shoulder at the front. Forward movement of a limb is named *protraction* (*extension*) and bending the limb is named *retraction* (*flexion*). The shoulder and hip joints are multiaxial and need to be stabilized for efficient forward movement. They must not fall in too far under the body or out too far away from the body. Different groups of muscles ensure this (see Figs. 5.2, 5.3 and 5.4).

Adductors: during normal activity these muscles prevent the limbs from falling outward and in dressage they are utilized to assist in lateral movements.

Abductors: during normal activity these muscles prevent the limbs from falling inward and in dressage they are utilized to assist in lateral movements.

These groups are very important, but are often overlooked. A masseur must be aware of their location and function. They are often found to be damaged or weak and lack of limb stability can cause a multitude of secondary problems.

A muscle never works as a single lone unit. All activity requires the balanced interaction of many groups. If a muscle or the joint it influences, or the ligaments of the joint, are damaged subtle differences within muscle actions take place. Muscles in areas often remote to the area of damage begin to act in uncharacteristic ways in an endeavour to complete movements as commanded and this leads to incorrect, uneconomic activity, often creating imbalance of force. In turn this leads to secondary problems.

A masseur should be aware of these factors. A visual increase in the contour of a muscle may be due to the overbuilding of the muscle or

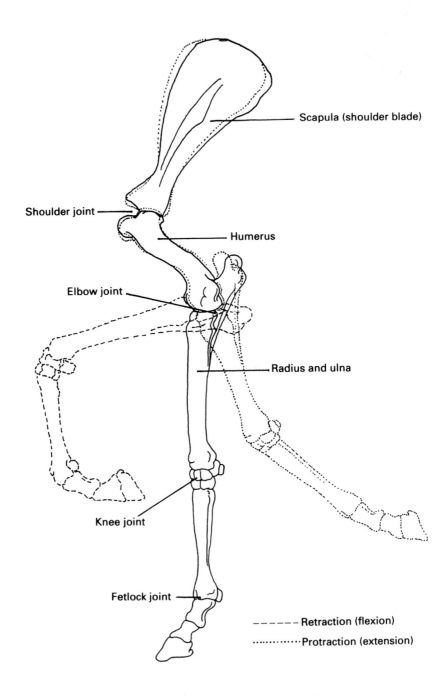

Fig. 5.2 The bone components of the shoulder and forelimb.

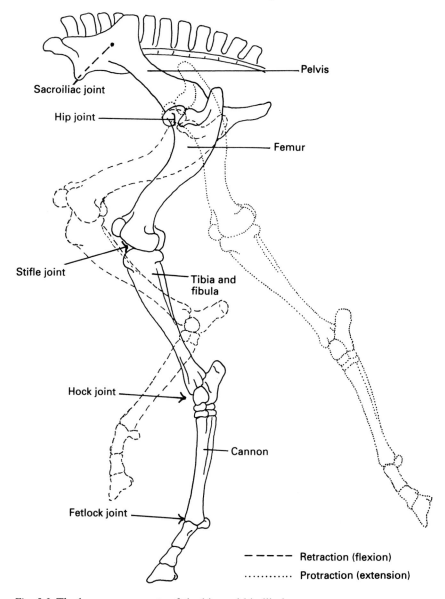

Sacroiliac joint

Hip joint

Pelvis

Femur

Stifle joint

Tibia and fibula

Hock joint

Cannon

Fetlock joint

– – – – – Retraction (flexion)

············· Protraction (extension)

Fig. 5.3 The bone components of the hip and hindlimb.

group rather than because of a local injury with apparent filling. For example, a horse with a problem in the off (right) hand limb and experiencing subclinical pain (a pain that does not cause obvious lameness) in the limb will hurry the movement of the near fore (left) limb, elevating the shoulder blade by using the trapezius muscle,

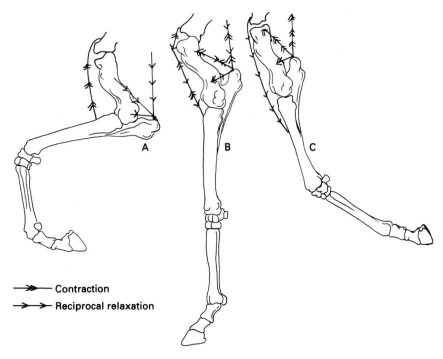

Fig. 5.4 Diagrammatic illustration of the interaction of the retractors and protractors of the shoulder.

normally a fixator rather than an active muscle. The resulting snatched action quickly transfers weight off the painful hind limb. The trapezius (sited at the top of the shoulder, just below the highest point of the withers) will accept the extra work but in doing so will increase in bulk and appear 'swollen' or larger than its fellow on the opposite side of the withers. Local massage to the 'swollen' shoulder will have no effect. The cause of pain, possibly in the opposite hind limb, must be found and addressed. Once again we are back to diagnosis. In this context the masseur must be familiar with:

- The location, nerve supply and actions of the muscles throughout the body.
- The muscles most subjected to stress for every known equine discipline.
- The directional flow and location of the main veins.
- The location of the lymphatic vessels.
- The techniques most suitable for general massage.

- The techniques most suitable for specific injuries common to horses.
- The ability to search for the cause of the problem should soreness or tension be encountered for no specific reason.
- The ability to visually assess the gaits of the horse as normal or abnormal. Careful assessment should include, if possible, watching the horse ridden. The tack, in particular the saddle fit should also be examined.
- The foot balance should be checked, as should the teeth.

The aims of the masseur should be to achieve a supple musculature enabling the horse to work in comfort. Masseurs and therapists are restorers – if you drop a piece of priceless porcelain you can have it restored. Drop it again, it will break once more. If you reduce muscle spasm or muscle pain without discovering the cause of the problem the moment the horse begins to work, if the problem is still present, the pain and stiffness will recur.

6 Hand Preparation and General Points for the Masseur

Your hands and their preparation

People rarely develop the full range of tactile senses available in their hands as our survival no longer depends on such levels of dexterity and touch appreciation. Who needs, like a tracker in African, an Aboriginal in Australia or a Dyak in the Malaysian jungle, to touch the ground to calculate the time elapsed since an animal passed or to touch a tree, plant, fruit to evaluate its condition? People who own and/or work with horses have developed some of the possible sensations as they 'feel legs', test for dehydration by pinching skin, run their hands over the coat to evaluate if it is starey or smooth, if there are small rain scald lumps, or to decide if a cracked heel is starting.

To massage successfully hand dexterity and touch sense need to be developed. This will not happen overnight – the art requires both time and practice, as do all forms of medicine. Remember, *medicine* is to *prevent* problems as well as to cure them.

Before starting on your horse ask a friend to act as your 'patient'. They will be able to tell you the sensations they receive from your hands – is it comfortable, do you exert too much pressure through the fingertips, does the thumb pinch, do you exert enough pressure or does it feel as though an ant is running over the skin, do the strokes achieve relaxation or create tension?

As well as using a human model for practice you must also prepare your hands. The muscle masses of the horse require greater hand strength to manipulate their bulk than do those of the average human.

Hand preparation
In Kim's game (an old-fashioned game) the child is blindfolded and asked to 'feel' a series of objects and then to describe their texture, shape, density and finally to guess and name each one. Try this as an exercise: the skin of an orange has a different texture to that of an

apple – does the orange have a 'starey coat' and the apple a 'good coat'? Feel two objects taken – one from the deep freeze and one from the refrigerator. The degree of 'cold' will differ. Appreciate this difference and then feel the outside of a mug of cooling liquid and register the sensations created. Everyone has a slightly different appreciation of feel and you must learn to retain the various sensations. What does muscle tension feel like to you? Does it feel 'hard' like pushing on a piece of wood, or does it feel like a stiff piece of leather? Everyone has to develop their own way of learning and retaining the sensations. There can be no set recipe stating that condition x feels like y. Once again we are up against the subtleties required to make a decision (diagnosis) before being able to choose an appropriate approach; a feature of all the complementary therapies.

Once you have mastered some of the tactile senses, suppleness and strength need to be addressed.

Exercises to strengthen and increase suppleness

All exercises should be performed in sets of seven.

Stretching for suppleness

Muscles that are warm and have a good stretch/recoil ability tire less easily. Remember that the joints and their ligaments are involved in any movement. The tendons to the fingers need to be considered. Although the hand has some very important little muscles, flexion (bending) and extension (straightening) are performed by the tendons of muscles sited in your forearms (see Fig. 6.1).

Exercise I

- Curl the fingers into a tight clench with the thumb under the fingers.
- Stretch to full extension and tense to achieve a shade more extension.
- Curl the fingers into a tight clench with the thumb over the fingers.
- Stretch as before.
- Spread the fingers as does a pianist stretching for an octave.
- Close and stretch again.
- With fingers clenched drop the wrist then lift up and press as far back above the horizontal as you can comfortably go.

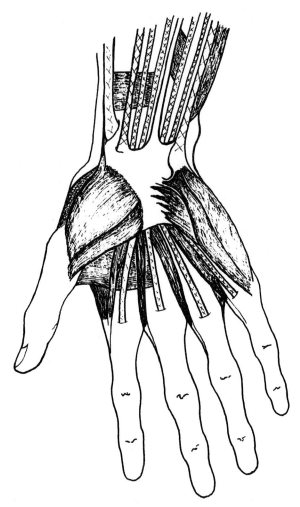

Fig. 6.1 The muscles and tendons of the palm.

After each part of Exercise I has been completed seven times, shrug and drop your shoulders until they too feel relaxed. In the early stages of learning to massage you will forget two things: firstly to breathe evenly, and secondly to keep your shoulders and body as relaxed as possible given the position you have to adopt to give massage. Shoulder tension fixes the upper part of the rib cage restricting upper chest movement and this in turn influences your breathing rhythm. Remember muscles require oxygen to function, and as you are using muscles in a new pattern and for long periods you must ensure you control your breathing. You must consider your own muscles if you are to avoid fatigue.

Strengthening the hands

To improve power and strength muscles need to work against an increased load so some form of resistance is required.

To strengthen the fingers a strong rubber band can be utilized to provide the external force. The nearer the band is placed to the tips of the fingers, the harder the work for the muscles. The middle (second) finger acts in an anchor and is mainly static when the index, second, ring and little fingers part and close. These actions are performed by the interossius muscles which lie between the five bones which form the frame for the hand.

Exercise II

This is to improve abduction in the interossius muscles.

- Using the middle (second) finger as the anchor place the rubber band tightly around the middle and index finger.
- Part the index finger from the middle finger, and at the end of the movement close index to middle.
- Repeat with ring and little fingers.

Exercise III

This is to improve adduction in the interossius muscles.

- Holding the rubber band in the other hand place it around the index finger while this finger is spread away from the middle finger.
- Close the index finger to middle finger against the resistance you apply via the rubber band.
- Repeat with ring and little fingers.

Exercise IV

This is to improve grasping or moulding.

- Take a squash, tennis or small ball that fits your hand in a manner that allows the fingers and thumb to grip the ball but without the fingertips touching.
- Squeeze and release.

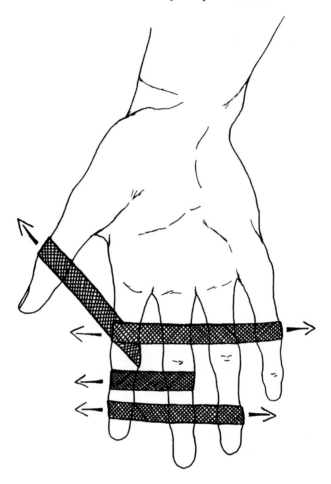

Fig. 6.2 Hand strengthening using a strong rubber band.

N.B.: Grip strengthening resistances are available in all sports equipment shops.

The thumb
The thumb is a highly specialized digit. The tip, in particular the ball, is endowed with a mass of sense receptors. It is capable of a series of highly complex movements and is able to work independently of the fingers as it has its own group of muscles sited at its base in the palm of the hand. These muscles form the thenar eminence. Move your own thumb around and see how many different directions and actions you can achieve.

Exercise V
This is to aid adduction in the thumb.

- Holding the rubber band in your other hand slip it over the ball of the thumb.
- Pull the thumb away from the index finger and keep the rubber band at stretch.
- Close the thumb back to the fingers.

Exercise VI
To help with abduction for the thumb.

- Slip the rubber band over the thumb and around the little finger while the thumb is against the index finger.
- Move the thumb away from the side of the index finger.

Exercise VII
This is for thumb opposition.

- Place the rubber band around the tip of the thumb with the thumb positioned at right angles to the palm of the hand.
- Holding the rubber band in your other hand move the thumb first to touch the base of the little finger, then touch the tip.
- Return to starting position.
- Repeat so the thumb touches base, then tip, of each of the other fingers.

N.B.: Each finger will bend in slightly to meet the thumb. This is normal and should be allowed to occur. Rotation of the thumb is achieved by the interaction of all the foregoing movements. Flexion and extension occur in the grasping exercise – Exercise IV.

Most people have a dominant hand, but successful massage requires both hands to be of the same strength, and for tactile sense and dexterity to be equal in both.

Hand use

The secret of success in massage is to learn more and more about your hands; explore with them, mentally file all pertinent sensations and activities. In the novice this requires a conscious appreciation of exactly what you want your hands to do, the ways in which you need to use feel, and what your hands tell you about the underlying tissues.

Running hands and fingertips over your 'friendly model' with your eyes closed will help you to learn the texture of superficial bone areas, limb contour and body angles. When you progress to the horse try to visualize the underlying muscles, their fibre direction and build in a 3D picture of the whole in your mind. Correctly administered massage should give as much satisfaction to the operator as it gives pleasure to the recipient.

Moulding the hands
Relaxation strokes require both hands to be moulded over the body, with the hands relaxed, yet firm, and exerting an *even* pressure.

Pressure
Variations in pressure will depend upon:

- The stroke or technique used
- The effect required
- The density of the underlying tissues
- The presence of superficial bone points

Rhythm

- Hand trembling, jerky movements, stops and starts will be resented and create tissue tension.
- Speed and pressure should be increased and decreased evenly in a smooth flowing manner.

Weight
Use your own body weight and movement rhythms as an aid. While your hands are the contact, exerting the expressive forces, the pressure is achieved by body rhythm, *not by tense hands*.

Finger sensation – touch
Tension is an acquired feature of muscles at rest. While maintaining sufficient *tone* to retain the upright position they should feel 'soft', rather like potter's clay.

Tension appreciation

Muscles 'guard' damaged areas, whether the damage is to bone, joint, ligament, tendon or the muscle itself. Increased tension will also occur if pain originates within an internal organ. Most horse owners have seen the tightness of the abdominal muscles in a horse with colic. Tension over the loins may be associated with the kidneys, so look for the cause of tension.

The feel of 'tense' or 'guarding' muscles has to be learnt and a meaningful comparison sought. What do you associate with the new sensation you have to teach your fingers to appreciate? As the fingertips become more sensitive so you will be able to feel the 'edges' of individual muscles, appreciate the presence of bone, calculate temperature and changes in surface moisture. All this information contributes to the diagnostic (deciding) process and every sensation change is pertinent. Even if you are massaging for health maintenance you may discover the small beginnings of a problem.

Problems

Perhaps your hands discover an area of tension which also feels warm and/or damp compared to neighbouring areas, and yet the rider has not reported a problem. A component within the mechanical unit must be at fault. Anatomical knowledge should tell you which joint or joints the muscle area influences, the nerve supply, and the bone levers. Any damage to tissue increases activity. Activity is a metabolic process which generates heat; excess heat is often lost through the porous skin as sweat. Your fingers have told you something is wrong so search for the *cause*. There is no problem without a cause and the problem cannot be solved unless the cause is addressed.

N.B.: Do not be fooled by areas of warmth which may have resulted from too tight a roller, the horse leaning against a wall, or the horse having been lying down, particularly if it was lying on a pile of droppings.

Finishing

After any type of massage always make a fuss of the horse and see it is comfortable. If rugged ensure the rugs are replaced correctly and rollers and or leg straps fitted properly. Finishing is as important as starting. Have a massage from an experienced masseur yourself and enjoy the pleasurable sensations. Then have a massage from a novice – you will appreciate the difference. Your ability to have experienced 'feel' yourself will help you to massage well.

General points for the masseur

As one of the aims of massage is relaxation the first approach to a new horse requires a slow tactful introduction.

(1)   Wear a kennel coat. It is a good idea to keep a clean one in your vehicle. There are two main reasons for this:
    (a)   A colt will not settle if you carry the smell of an in-season filly on your clothes.
    (b)   Some of your clients may be ill or their yard may have a virus, and an attempt at hygiene will be appreciated by owners.
(2)   Wear shoes or boots strong enough to give your feet some protection in case your foot gets trodden on as the horse moves.
(3)   It is preferable to work on a horse in its own box. The horse should wear a head collar. If the animal is restless and needs restraint it is best to use a long rope looped through the tie ring with the free end held in the operator's non-operative hand. Occasionally massage is painful and if the horse is tied and pulls back suddenly it may, in the future, associate restraint with pain.
(4)   Never use a twitch or other severe restraint. The animal's muscles will tense and it will be impossible to work.
(5)   Make certain there is nothing you can trip over if you have to move suddenly.
(6)   Remember that every horse will have a different level of tolerance.
(7)   Every horse will react in a different manner to the various techniques.
(8)   Never underestimate the rapidity with which a horse can react: if you become complacent you will get hurt.
(9)   Start your massage session by feeling the neck to find the area that causes the horse to lean on you and 'ask for more'. Pleasure is often accompanied by the horse trying to reciprocate, and it may attempt to chew your shoulder.
(10) Work towards the ears and pull and massage them. This will encourage further relaxation and increase confidence.
(11) When the horse is used to you begin to work other muscle groups, all the time feeling for increased tension in the tissues.
(12) Work the muscle groups associated with the horse's discipline, choosing the technique appropriate to the area.

(13) If possible massage before exercise.
(14) Try to work in parallel to the lie of the underlying tissue fibres and also to the venous and/or lymphatic return.
(15) Follow work on painful areas by work on areas you know the horse will enjoy.
(16) Start and finish each session with comforting effleurage.
(17) Do not hurry – a good massage takes around 45 minutes.
(18) Massage for specific conditions should, whenever possible, include a general body rub.
(19) A milk crate makes a very useful platform if you are not tall enough to work in comfort from the ground.

7 Massage Techniques, Effects and Uses

Strokes – techniques, effects and uses

Massage strokes are varied. Few people use their hands in an exactly similar manner, but this does not matter.

Basic rules
If the coat lie allows, work in the direction of venous return. Of the main collecting areas for venous blood and lymphatic fluid the two most readily available are on the inner side of the elbow and in the groin, and it is perfectly possible to direct strokes *towards* these areas.

- Start and finish with effleurage.
- Do not cause pain.
- If you increase tension rather than reduce it, change technique.
- If you use oils or liniments make certain that:
  (a) the horse is not allergic to them, and
  (b) you do not 'blister' the area.
- When massaging locally make certain the skin and underlying tissues move as one. 'Skin slipping' (skin sliding over underlying tissues) will create a local blister.
- In all cases with tendon or leg problems work over the bulbs of the heels, in association with localized work for the problem tissue.
- A general massage with strokes directed to the muscle groups always involved in any activity and also those required to undertake extra work, dependent on the discipline, if given *before* exercise, improves performance.
- A general massage, strokes directed, in the main, to the muscle groups used during activity will assist recovery and aid in lessening post-exertion fatigue.
- Consider the direction of the muscle fibres and work *with* them,

not across them, unless treating a condition necessitating cross fibre work.

● If only using one hand, the free hand should be positioned on the body mass to act as a 'support contact'.

Effleurage

In general, this technique involves both hands. They are moulded over the body contours, and contact is established throughout the entire surface of palm, thumb and fingers. The hands may lie beside each other, one behind the other or be moulded around a limb, one above the other.

In massage manuals, the stroke is described as a long straight push with the hands exerting the effective pressure as they are moved *away* from the body of the masseur. A light contact must be maintained as the hands return to their starting position.

However the most effective effleurage stroke may need to be *towards* the masseur, rather than away, because of the growth direc-

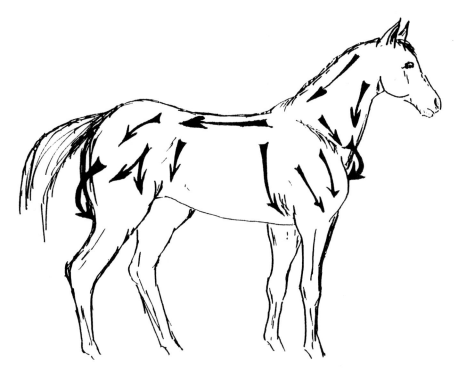

Fig. 7.1 Stroke direction for effleurage.

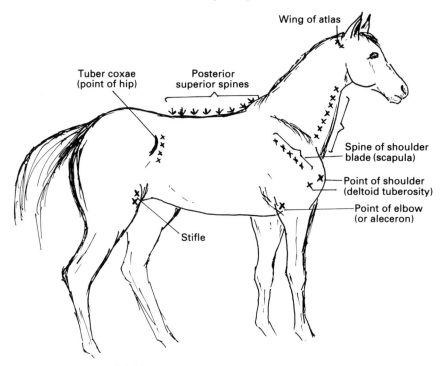

Fig. 7.2 Avoid superficial boney areas.

tions of a horse's coat, and the fact that two available venous and lymphatic collecting sites lie in the elbow and groin areas.

Pressure should be firm but not heavy until the animal begins to relax. Pressure can be increased as relaxation occurs. The final depth of compression should relate to tissue mass and location.

After each completed stroke, the direction and starting and finishing points are varied and strokes redirected until the whole area has been worked over. The strokes should be performed in an even rhythmic manner.

Start and finish all massage sessions with effleurage as it has the following effects:

- Relaxation
- Reduction of tension
- Reduction of pain
- Assistance to venous and lymphatic flow
- Due to the influence on venous return the arterial delivery is also enhanced which 'warms' the tissues.

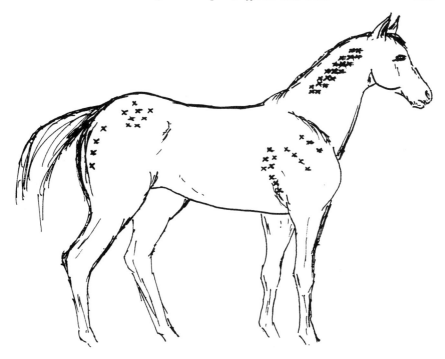

Fig. 7.3 Muscle mass areas suitable for kneading.

Kneading

In general this is a single handed technique (see Fig. 7.4). The purpose is to effect a deep compression followed by reduced compression. The technique is used to affect deep sited problems in large masses of muscle.

The working hand is clenched in a loose fist, and the backs of the fingers and the knuckles are positioned over the pertinent area. The movement is first directed downward deep into the muscle mass. When both depth and required compression have been attained the fist should roll in a slightly angled and upward manner to release compression. The movement sequence can be likened to that used when 'scooping out' deep frozen ice cream.

The technique demands some twisting (rotation) of the wrist and shoulder of the operative arm. As one hand tires introduce the other hand.

Kneading has the following effects:

● Compression of deep circulatory vessels local to and within the tissue

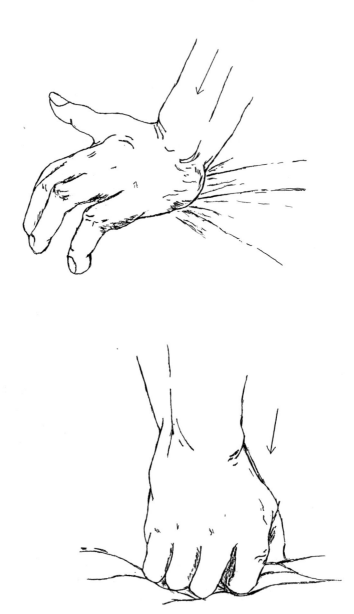

Fig. 7.4 Kneading or deep compression using the heel of the hand or knuckles.

- Stress/stretching of deep scarring
- Pain reduction
- Haematoma breakdown

Wringing

The technique is double handed. The skin and underlying tissue are picked up, *not by the fingers* but within the *palm and fingers* of first one hand and then the other. As one hand lifts and pulls upward so the second must lower. As the two hands pass each other a slight 'twist' is introduced, thus the tissues between the two hands are subjected to a slight rotational stress. The movement can be compared to that performed when hand-wringing laundry. This has the following effects:

- Compression of local circulatory vessels
- Stretching of tight skin and underlying tissue
- The stretching improves elasticity within muscle tissue

N.B.: Remember to work so that the stretch is parallel to muscle fibre lie.

Percussion or hacking

This is a two handed technique. The little finger sides of both hands are placed just above the area to be treated, then by twisting (rotating) first one and then the other forearm, the relaxed sides of the hands and little fingers achieve an alternating, short, sharp contact with the underlying tissue. The effects are:

- Vibratory
- Mild stimulation of underlying muscle
- Stimulation of surface vessels

In the human the technique is used to assist drainage in chest conditions. Because of the horse's inability to 'cough up' mucus from the lungs it is doubtful if this effect will assist problems within equine lungs.

Skin rolling

A double handed finger technique. A flap of skin is picked up between the fingers and thumbs. It is then gently pushed away using thumb pressure against slightly restraining fingers and as the hands move away from the body, so one area of skin 'rolls' into another.

The skin can then be rolled back toward the masseur with the fingers pushing and thumbs restraining. At the end of a movement, release the tissue and relocate the hands as required. The technique can be likened to the surge and collapse of a sea swell. The effects are:

- Stretching contracted areas of skin tissue
- Improvement of skin circulation
- Stimulation of skin components

Friction
Friction is a local technique when either the thumb or one finger, usually the index reinforced by the second, is used to perform a deep penetrating movement. This may be *circular* or *transverse* across the line of the underlying tissue fibres.

Circular. Place the thumb or finger over the area and work in a series of small circular movements around or over the selected area (see Fig. 7.5). The effects are:

- Hyperaemia
- Stretching of scar tissue
- Breakdown of adhesions
- Pain reduction

Transverse. This is performed most effectively with the tip of the index finger reinforced by the second finger. The tip is placed over the fibres of the structure to be worked upon (the thumb can be used for a support). The tip of the finger is moved in a transverse manner across and back over the damaged or scarred area. To be effective deep pressure should be applied.

N.B.: The fingertip must *not* 'skin slip' – the underlying skin should move as one with the fingertip. The effects of this are:

- To create a local hyperaemia
- To break down scar tissue
- To break down an organized haematoma
- To break down adhesions
- To stimulate acupressure points thereby relieving pain and/or muscle spasm

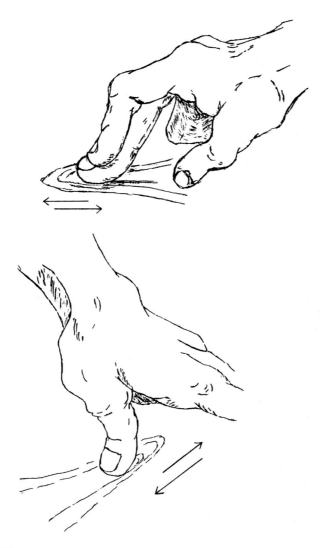

Fig. 7.5 Finger positioning for friction massage.

Once again we find interconnection between the 'natural therapies' of massage and acupressure.

Finger massage

The fingers can be used effectively without the palm of the hand. Small muscles, for example rectus capitus, and tissues sited in confined areas such as behind the knee would be difficult to massage using the entire hand. Similarly tendons, ligaments and the bulbs of the heels can be massaged with greater accuracy with the fingertips.

The hand techniques can be modified but as the pressure applied will be to a small area care must be taken to massage rather than to friction.

As with all techniques the chosen approach needs to be appropriate both for the result required and *the state of the tissue.*

Ice massage

Recent injury responds to cold application in the following ways:

- For approximately the first 15 minutes of application closing or constriction of local blood vessels occurs.
- There is decreased activity in local tissue reducing immediate oxygen requirement.
- Thermo-regulators (sensors) record and monitor the drop in temperature.
- As the ambient tissue temperature drops to an unacceptable low the arterial circulation is alerted and a surge of 'warming' blood is dispatched.

N.B.: This safety mechanism will *not* operate if the temperature remains sub-zero for a long period as the sensors *cease to record.*

Ice techniques can be employed for large areas by placing ice cubes in a plastic bag (hand held size), then massaging using a circular movement. The ice pack should be moved over the traumatized area for approximately 5–10 minutes.

Local application to a small area

An individual ice cube can be rubbed over recent trauma in a circular manner. A supply of ice cubes with a 'stick' handle (iced lolly containers come in suitable sizes) kept in a deep freeze ready for trauma application is a useful tool.

Connective tissue massage

Each individual muscle is partitioned from its fellows by an outer sleeve of connective tissue. Look at a half leg of lamb at the next opportunity. You can plainly see fine white lines arranged around the masses of the red flesh of the muscles. The white lines are the muscle *sleeves* or *sheaths.* If you try to detach one mass and its sleeve or sheath from another you will discover that adjacent sheaths are inter-connected, one to the other, hence the term *connective tissue*. Con-nective tissue massage is directed to these areas.

Connective tissue does not contain many elastic components. Should a muscle suddenly increase in bulk as a result of exercise, the connective tissue sheath may not immediately stretch to accommodate the volume increase. Stretch receptors will then record pain and muscle metabolism is hampered as the muscle attempts to work to increased demand and painful, ineffective contraction will result.

It is *sometimes* possible to relieve pain and stretch the affected connective tissue by directing a deep friction based massage along the lines of the connective tissue bands.

This is impossible without an extensive knowledge of the anatomical arrangement of the muscles.

Choice of techniques
The selection of strokes or techniques (either mechanical or hand) must rest with the masseur, as will the decision to incorporate passive stretches. Conformation, fitness, rider weight, equine discipline and tissue trauma, all need to be considered before deciding on an effective regime.

Each discipline demands certain predominant muscular activity. The muscles of the dressage horse work mainly in middle and inner range, while the muscles of the thoroughbred racehorse are expected to work through all ranges but with great demands upon the outer range. The polo pony and cattle horse are required to perform movements stressing the hocks with the muscle activity mainly in the inner range.

The variables of muscle activity can be more clearly appreciated by watching horses performing athletically and linking anatomical knowledge to movement. In cases where muscle trauma has occurred, a video (if available) will always help assess possible problems and their sites. If athletes are filmed as they perform and if their falls and performance are recorded, study of the films will nearly always pin-point problem areas.

Effects of massage

Massage is the art of rubbing with external stimulation applied via the operator's hands affecting deeper structures. Even local massage will affect the 'whole'. Once again we find a medical method with a holistic approach which originated centuries ago.

Pain relief

If a child falls and rushes to its parent crying, the immediate reaction is to ask 'where does it hurt?' and then rub the area. Everyone does this instinctively, whether it is their child or themselves who is experiencing pain.

Science has shown that rubbing an area causes the pain control system of a body to release pain killing chemicals manufactured by and within the body. The body has its own ability to make opiates. These are stored and released (when needed) in response to commands.

Relaxation

The body is supplied with myriads of 'sense receptors'. These are specialist nerve endings which receive, record, document, emit commands and transmit messages from all the body components.

Science has shown that cyclical repetition of many of the external stimuli experienced, or available in daily life, can temporarily change the advance recording mechanisms in certain sense receptors, thus reducing their activity in areas of tension. Relaxation or reduction of tension is secondary to some types of massage, and tension relaxation has several 'knock on' effects (see Fig. 7.6).

Improved venous and lymphatic fluid flow

The veins and lymphatic vessels are the major components of the return vessel network (see Fig. 7.7). Venous blood loaded with waste and lymph (the fluid component of the system which is primarily concerned with combating any form of invasion of the body, be it toxic, bacterial or from a virus) are both slow fluid movers. Both lymphatic flow and venous blood flow can be assisted by massage.

In order to prevent blood back-flow the veins are fitted with small non-return cusp-like valves. These are sited, rather like locks on a canal, at regular intervals within the hollow interior of the veins. Compression in the form of long, deep, smooth strokes, applied in the direction the blood returns, aids the passage of venous blood from section to section within the vein particularly in areas where there is an absence of contracting muscle.

The lymphatic flow has no pumping organ like the heart. Movement within the system is not clearly understood and it is doubtful if

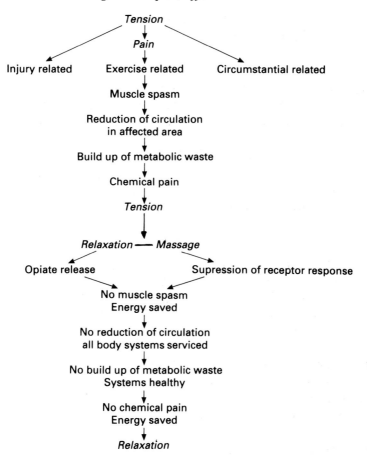

Fig. 7.6 Effects of tension and relaxation.

the extent of the system in the horse has been fully documented in the current anatomy books. It is suggested that the compression and relaxation effected by massage will affect lymph movement. The flow is considered to run in parallel to that within the veins and many lymph vessels lie in conjunction with the veins.

Local massage
A hyperaemia or increased local circulatory flow occurs secondary to the compressive and/or irritant effects created. This increase, within local circulation, will ensure both increased delivery of cells to aid recovery, and the removal of trauma debris, a particularly useful effect in areas of restricted circulatory flow.

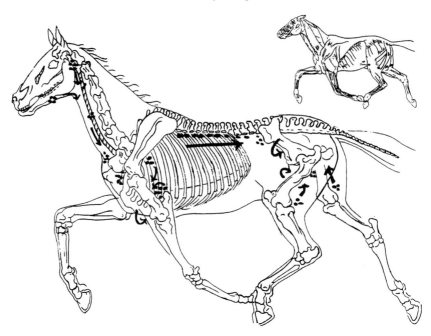

Fig. 7.7 Sites of lymph nodes (*after Sissons and Grossman*). The lymphatic system of the horse as described in anatomy books makes no mention of lymph vessels or centres in the limbs. It is presumed that the system lies adjacent to the venous system.

Circulatory increase, even in a local area affects the entire system. Circulation cannot be hyperactive in one area only, so although the effect of any local increase may only achieve a minimal general effect there will be an overall response due to the intricate interlinking of all the body systems.

Relaxation and the associated improved venous and lymphatic flow, be it local or general, also affect the whole body. The circulatory system as described in Chapter 1 infiltrates every part of the whole. It services the brain, central and peripheral nervous systems, the bones, the soft tissues, all the organs, the skin, in fact *every* component that requires an adequate blood flow. Thus any assistance which *does not require the body to expend energy* is of the greatest value in the maintenance of health.

Obviously activity increases circulatory movement, *but* activity requires energy, energy gives rise to waste, waste requires removal, energy needs to be replenished, replenishment leads to further activity, and so describing the effects of massage as being only 'relaxation, pain reduction, increased lymph and venous return' is inadequate as these four factors have dramatic effects on the whole.

Good grooming has a massaging effect, many of the syce (grooms) in India, Malaysia and in the Middle East groom using their hands rather than brushes. Their charges revel in the hand contact, their coats shine and their muscles are supple.

Strapping with a strapping pad is a form of generalized compression and relaxation, *but* it is an *active* process needing energy with the muscles contracting beneath the impact of the pad. The straw wisp, a part of a grooming kit until straw became too short to plait, was used in a manner resembling effleurage.

8 Massage Equipment and Routines

Massage equipment

There is no substitute for hands, however hand massage is time-consuming and very exhausting when done correctly.

Massage machines

Massage machines do not massage – they vibrate creating a compression/relaxation effect upon the underlying tissues with the following effects:

- Constant vibrations delivered at a constant cyclical repetition are known to evoke a temporary analgesia within the tissues treated (*pain reduction*).

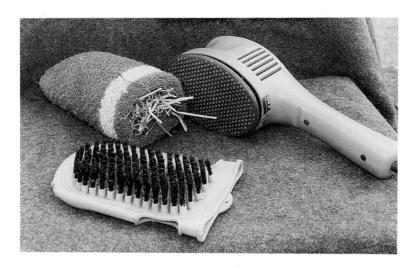

Plate 8.1 An electric vibrator and two massage gloves.

- The compression/relaxation will affect the vessels immediately below the applicator ('knock on' effects of *very mild circulatory influence*).
- Pain relief *reduces local muscle spasm* allowing normal circulatory flow to re-establish.
- Resumption of circulation *enhances muscle activity* and/or *healing*.

Mechanical massagers which are effective for the equine body mass are powered electrically and need a mains supply. Some are designed to be hand-held, and some comprise large pads formed to mould to the contours of the horse's back.

Technique

- Turn on the machine in the box to accustom the horse to the noise.
- Turn off the machine and rub it over an area of the neck which you know will relax the horse.
- Turn on the machine and move around gently over the neck, working over the body to reach the area to be treated.
- Even when the horse is accustomed to the machine and the noise, use the same starting technique – horses, like humans, have good and bad days!

Massage gloves

There are several massage gloves on the market. The operator's hand and fingers fit into a mitten, often made of flexible synthetic rubber-like material, the palm side of which may be ridged, or covered in small raised 'bushes' like the soles of some golf shoes, or have minute cone-like extensions.

The most useful are designed for the human rather than the horse. They are called 'bath mittens' and they enclose the hand providing a useful, light, easily moulded, slightly roughened surface giving a good grip and comfortable feel. They are particularly useful for gaining an animal's confidence, supposedly because the sensation must be similar to that experienced if the animal rubs against tree bark.

Technique

- Effleurage type strokes are best suited to massage gloves.
- Incorporate glove massage with hand massage.

Underwater massage

The lower end of horses' legs do not have an adequate circulatory return as the veins in the lower third of the legs are without the valves whose function is to ensure a one-way no return flow. The lower third of the limb is dependent on the pumping actions of the frog. This action is not fully efficient unless the horse has a correctly balanced foot. The frog, if able to function, aids fluid return from both the foot and fetlock area. Frog action is aided by the movements of the sole of the foot, and these movements are also dependent upon foot balance, shape, health and trim. Pooling of fluid is all too often present just above the fetlocks. Submersion of the limb, if possible to above the knee or hock, in cold agitated water helps reduce such filling. The moving water compresses and relaxes tissue and this in turn aids the 'shunt' of venous blood. The cold also has a thermal knock on effect. As the limb temperature drops to below the ambient set by the body's thermal centre, specialist receptors signal the need for a temperature rise. The response is a sudden arterial blood shunt within the deep limb vessels, and this in turn increases local pressure with a further knock on effect within the veins associated with the particular arterial complex.

Wellie boots
Large rubberized boots, one for each leg, are attached to a motor by a pipe. The horse is persuaded to stand with his leg or legs inside the boots, and water is introduced by a hose. Crushed ice can also be added for extra cooling. When the boots are filled the motor can be switched on. Air which agitates the water is delivered at the toe of the boot via a pipe and non-return valve.

There is no danger of damaging the horse as the boots are pliable. They merely fall over spilling the water if the horse decides to evacuate.

Jacuzzi tub
This employs the same principle as the boots – air agitated water. The disadvantage is that the horse must put both feet into the same tub. The advantage is that the tub is larger than the boot, more stable and does not have to be emptied and refilled at each session.

Underwater massage is useful for filled legs, but hand massage should precede water massage.

Technique for underwater massage

- Persuade the horse to place a leg in the tub or boot.
- Fill with water.
- Let the horse stand and relax.
- Add crushed ice if required.
- Turn on the water agitator, and run it for ten to fifteen minutes.
- Dry off leg.

N.B.: If the horse objects to standing in the water-filled container, hosing the legs first will nearly always achieve the desired result. Horses with wet legs are less reluctant to stand in water.

Positioning the horse for massage

- The horse must be in a box with bedding on a non-slip floor.
- You must be able to reach every part of the horse both safely and in a manner allowing you to use your body weight to achieve stroke pressure.
- To reach the back you may need height. A milk crate is a useful mobile stand, the disadvantage being it only offers a small base. A firm 'side' to the horse's bed may offer a better base area.
  (The milk crate is also useful as a seat for leg techniques.)

Restraint

- The horse should wear a head collar.
- Tying with a quick release restraint may be necessary in the early sessions.
- If possible achieve a state of trust that allows the horse to stand free. He can then move if *hurt* or *irritated* by you.

Starting

- Allow the horse to smell your hands. If you are using a gel or oil let the animal smell it.
- Run your hands over the neck, back and quarters to let the animal get used to the feel of your hands.
- Depending upon the type of massage required (general or specific) you should have decided upon the approach and techniques needed after hearing the problems being exhibited, i.e. stiff on the

left rein, unable to achieve an outline, won't break from the stalls, etc.

● For other than a general toning massage, you must have a specific diagnosis.

● When the animal is used to your presence and the feel and smell of your hands, it is time to begin a planned session.

N.B.: Anyone can be wrong. If your plan does not seem to be effective, think again. It takes courage to admit to mistakes but it earns respect.

Massage routines

There can be no set massage routines or recipes, each horse's requirements will vary. There are many factors to take into account: the equine discipline, the rider's report describing the 'feel' experienced while riding, muscle contour, and details of the accident sustained should all help to alert the masseur to areas which may require special attention.

The masseur should also be aware of the muscles subjected to unusual stress in each of the differing equine activities and pay special attention to those muscles.

Most often overlooked are the muscle groups concerned with adduction. In the forelimb the muscles lie at the base of the chest and continue backward between the forelegs to approximately a hand span behind the girth – these are known as the pectorals. In the hindlimb the muscles lie on the inner side of the upper part of the thigh stretching up into the groin. Vastus medialis, intermedius, sartorius and gracilis are all adductors. The last two are long strap-like muscles, and both are partially inserted into the medial patella ligament aiding stability within the stifle joint. The ligament is often highly sensitive to palpation and it is for this reason that it has been suggested that the ligament be considered within a general massage routine.

Once again, as discussed in all previous sections, success or failure rests upon an adequate assessment (*diagnosis*). In the case of massage this assessment or diagnosis will be made by the masseur, enabling the approach most appropriate for each individual to be selected.

N.B.: Remember tissue is alive, and conditions change continuously. The suggestions in this book are based upon experience; they are *not* hard and fast rules.

Stretches incorporated in a massage routine must also be selected carefully.

A routine for effleurage (refer to Fig. 7.1)

A pre-exercise/competition general massage using the effleurage technique will enhance muscle activity. If your horse tends to wander around the box as you try to massage it must be restrained by being racked up. It is preferable for the animal to wear a head collar and to leave a short lead rope hanging free lest sudden restraint is necessary.

If possible, plan your learning massage sessions when the yard is quiet and there is little chance of being disturbed. Once your horse is accustomed to the pleasurable sessions it will usually arrange itself comfortably and wait for you to start no matter what is happening around you both.

Neck and shoulders

(1) Position yourself by or just forward of the horse's shoulder, facing the tail on whichever side of the horse you feel most comfortable.

(2) Place your hands flat just behind the poll, fingers pointing upward towards the top of the neck. Pull your hands slowly and firmly down from the top of the neck toward the withers. Remove the hands and replace at your original starting point. Repeat several times until you feel the muscles relax (soften).

(3) Direct the next pair of parallel strokes from poll downward to the base of the neck, pulling the hands down. Repeat until relaxation occurs.

(4) Move slightly forward until you are positioned almost in front of and facing the horse with its head over one or other of your shoulders. Direct the strokes from withers to the front of the chest by pulling the hands toward you. Repeat until relaxation occurs.

(5) Place your hands on either side of the withers and direct the stroke down toward the elbows of the animal. If you cannot reach easily work first on one side, then on the other, moving your body to the side upon which you are working.

As you massage reposition your body slowly, trying to maintain a rhythm in tune with the strokes. Try not to tense your shoulders (you will tire quickly if you tense) and do not forget to breathe (people tend to hold their breath as they concentrate!). If your horse is very tall you may have to adapt, working first on one side of the animal and then on the other. Using both hands, one on either side of the animal is not only economic time-wise, but more beneficial physiologically. Effective warming of underlying muscle and relaxation normally occurs after ten to fifteen strokes.

The back

(1) Position yourself just in front of the quarters on whichever side of the horse *you* feel most comfortable. (If the horse is very tall stand on a milk crate.) Lean slightly forward and place a hand on either side of the animal's withers close to the spine, with the hands positioned so that the fingers point toward the animal's head. Draw the hands slowly toward your body, exerting an even pressure. Repeat several times before going on to the next stage.

(2) Moving the hands apart and repeating the strokes, gradually work further away from the centre of the back. The longissimus muscle stretches from withers to quarters and is approximately the width of one hand to two hands span, depending on the size of the horse, from the middle of the back outward.

Repeat as for stage 1 until the entire muscle in length and breadth has been massaged.

The quarters

(1) Stay in the same position as when massaging the back, but turn to face the tail. Place a hand on either side of the top of the quarters with fingers pointing away from your body, and push the hands away toward the root of the tail.

The flanks and muscles at the top of each hind leg running up to the dock (hamstrings) are better massage by first standing on the near side and then repositioning on the off side. To work directly behind any horse, however quiet, *must be done with great care!*

Near side quarter

(1) Face the quarters and place your left hand on the loins for support contact. Place the right hand at the top of the quarters just below the jumpers bump (tuber sacralae) with the fingers

pointing away from your body. Push the hand down and back toward the dock, then onward and downward to finish the stroke on the inner side of the second thigh (gaskin).

(2) Place the hand below the point of the hip (tuber coxae), fingers pointing towards the stifle, and draw the hand downward ending one stroke angling forward toward the stifle. The following stroke should be angled toward the back of the second thigh.

(3) Place the hand forward of the point of the hip (tuber coxae), fingers pointing upward, and *very gently* exerting a firm but light pressure draw the hand down toward the stifle.

N.B.: This is often resented. If this is the case abandon the stroke. Repeat the series on the offside quarter working with the left hand, and using the right hand as the support contact.

Once you are adept, the total massage should take between 10–20 minutes.

A precompetition massage is best given just before the animal begins its normal precompetition exercise warm-up.

Passive stretches are best given after massage, as they are designed to increase joint range as well as to increase muscle suppleness. They are *not* essential on the day of the competition. Their best use would seem to be during the period of fitness work given pre-season whatever the discipline.

Post-exercise or competition
Most horses are groomed after being ridden, even if only hacked out. Strenuous exercise, whatever the reason, fatigues muscles and a massage given approximately two hours after exertion, when the horse has dried off, had a drink and eaten, will reduce the chances of stiffness the following day. Five to eight minutes effleurage should be given first, and then followed by techniques specific for the muscle groups involved in the specific discipline. Techniques suitable for the main superficial muscle groups are as follows.

(1) Rectus capitus   } Gentle finger massage
(2) Brachiocephalicus
(3) Supraspinatus   } Knead gently
(4) Infraspinatus
(5) Triceps   Deep kneading
(6) Pectorals   Knead gently

(7)	Trapezius	Knead
(8)	Longissimus	Gentle kneading. The muscle mass is often grossly diminished in horses in poor condition, and finger massage should be used.
(9)	Gluteus medius	Deep kneading
(10)	Tensor fascia lata	Knead/finger massage
(11)	Biceps femoris	Knead/wring/finger massage
(12)	Semi-tendonosis	Knead/wring/finger massage
(13)	Gastrocnemius	Finger massage
	Medial patella ligament	Finger massage.

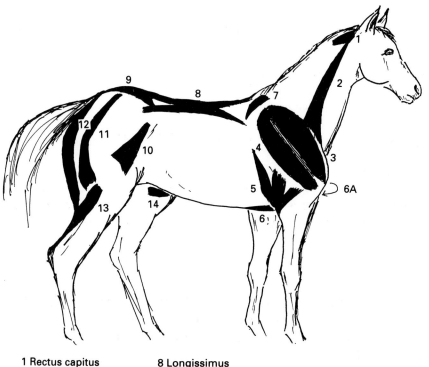

1 Rectus capitus
2 Brachiocephalicus
3 Supraspinatus
4 Infraspinatus
5 Triceps
6 and 6A Pectoralis
7 Trapezius
8 Longissimus
9 Gluteus medius
10 Tensor fascia lata
11 Biceps femoris
12 Semitendonosis
13 Gastrocnemius
14 Medial patella ligament

Fig. 8.1 General massage to improve performance.

Close with effleurage. Time required is approximately 45 minutes.

As a general rule, work a specific technique on one side of the animal and then move to the other side. This is more relaxing than 'doing over' one side and then starting on the other.

Regard the horse as a whole. Keep the horse warm.

Stretches

Passive stretches should be performed *after* the tissues to be stretched have been warmed by massage. At the first assessment *all* the stretches should be performed and the 'end feel' and range of each assessed. Those that require attention can be noted and incorporated in future massage sessions.

Specific conditions of the limbs

Massage for tendon and lower leg problems.

I Tenosynovitis

- This condition occurs when the lubricant sheath of the tendon becomes inflamed.
- Heat and swelling are present.
- The fingers and thumb will often feel a 'grating sensation' in the underlying tissue if the leg is picked up, the swollen area held between finger and thumb and then the fetlock flexed and extended.

Technique

- Finger massage in the direction of the tendon fibres, moving the skin and sheath as one upon the main tendon.
- Massage the 'parent' muscle at the back of the limb.
- Stretch knee and fetlock as one.
- Treat daily for 15–20 minutes.
- Ice is useful – massage with a cube.
- Use protraction stretches.

II Tendon rupture

Rupture of tendon fibres is unfortunately all too common. It has various causes. In order to increase speed the limb levers, in particular the cannon bone, have been lengthened by selective breeding, thus the flexor tendons are under greater strain during extension and this is a possible cause of tendon failure.

- Heat accumulates in the core of the tendons during activity and rapidly reaches a critical level, creating fragile tissue which may rupture spontaneously.
- Imbalance of foot creates a torque stressing the vertical lie of fibres incorrectly.
- The horse may strike into himself or be struck into by another horse if racing.
- Heat and swelling are present.
- The tendon may bow.

Technique

- Apply local ice massage in the early stages, treating twice daily for, if possible, 15–20 minutes.
- Apply local friction massage as the swelling (oedema) resolves.
- *Do not stretch until veterinary agreement has been given*
- Always massage:
    - The undamaged areas above and below the lesion.
    - The bulbs of the heels to assist venous return.
    - The parent muscle.
- Treat daily for 10–21 days. Time required is approximately 15–20 minutes.

III Suspensory ligament

Technique

- Massage as for II Tendon rupture.

IV Check ligament strain

Technique

- Massage as for II Tendon rupture.
- There is no parent muscle associated with either ligament.
- Treat the leg above and below the lesion.
- *Do not stretch until veterinary agreement has been given.*

V Carpal tunnel strain

Technique

- Treat as for II Tendon rupture.
- Use both protraction shoulder stretches.

VI Sesamoid bruising

The sesamoid bones have a very poor circulatory supply. The bruising is usually caused by connection with a passing hoof in flight. It is bone bruising with the haemorrhage lying between the bone and its over-lying periostium.

Technique

- Massage with ice immediately (if possible).
- Instruct the owner to perform ice massage hourly for 5–10 minutes at *least* every two hours for 24 hours.
- Follow with finger massage to the area over the bruising
  - to the fetlock
  - behind the pastern
  - in the bulbs of the heels.

The aims of treatment in Conditions 1– VI are to:

- Improve venous return thus improving general circulatory flow
- Control and reduce oedema
- Prevent adhesions

The neck and back

Horses who fall when competing, get cast in the box, slip on a road, or lose, for any reason, their normal four limb balance will twist neck and/or back as they make frantic efforts to regain their feet. The exertions will stress the normal balanced alignment of one or more areas of the back, the neck or both.

The trauma areas are easily located by palpation. Carefully palpate the entire length of neck from ears to withers and then the back from withers to croup. Incorporate the neck/back stretch routines as an aid to the location of the areas of trauma. Increased tension will be felt, with the muscle 'hardening' to touch.

Technique

- First use effleurage for pain relief and relaxation.
- Follow with local finger techniques to the areas assessed as being painful.
- Use general effleurage to close.
- Incorporate stretches *immediately* to prevent adhesions.
- Time allowed will depend upon the extent of the problem, but 15–20 minutes is the minimum.

Bruising

Bruising is usually caused by the horse colliding with an obstacle while competing or being kicked.

A tiresome bruise may occur as the horse enters or leaves its box. This can be caused both by rushing and being too close to one or other side of the doorframe. The point of the hip (tuber coxae) hits the doorframe and can be severely bruised by the contact. As there are a number of very important muscle attachments in this area pain on all movements of the hind limb will result.

Technique

- Ice massage the bruised area as speedily as is possible.
- Follow with general effleurage to surrounding areas for 15–20 minutes. Do this twice, if possible, on day 1.
- After 24 hours, massage surrounding muscles using a general routine.
- Follow by massaging the perimeter of the area of tension/bruising with the fingers, working toward the centre of the area.
- Repeat the general massage to the surrounding muscle masses.
- Treat daily until the bruise resolves.
- Time required is approximately 20–30 minutes.
- Follow with appropriate passive stretches.

Torn muscle

Tears within the architecture of a muscle occur if the fibres, often in a state of fatigue, are overstretched. The tears may occur near the origin of the muscle, in the main body (belly) of the muscle, or at the musculo-tendinous junction where muscle fibres begin to change their structural pattern to regroup as tendon. The amount of discomfort exhibited will depend upon the number of fibres involved and the secondary side effects.

When the muscle fibres tear chemical activators are released into the tissue spaces adjacent to the tear. Their presence acts as a signal and the circulatory supply to the area is increased immediately.

Unfortunately the body responses tend to overreact and an excess of fluids arrive only to accumulate in and around the damaged area. The increase in pressure causes pain and reduces the functional ability of local undamaged tissue.

Signs of a muscle tear

- Pain on palpation
- Local heat
- Swelling
- Reduced activity of the muscle
- A change in the way of going, often almost imperceptible

Technique

- Immediate ice application.
- Ice massage around and over the area of damage 24–48 hours after injury.
- Effleurage working toward the elbow or groin.
- As the swelling decreases (timing will depend upon the severity of the tear) begin to use the appropriate techniques, massaging daily until a normal pain-free state is achieved.
- Use the appropriate passive stretches to avoid scarring after 48–56 hours.

Specialist disciplines and their requirements

Competitive sport requires specialist training routines. In the human athlete the biomechanics of each discipline have been studied and exercise routines to meet the particular needs of each type of sport have been developed.

Equine sports medicine is in its infancy. The firing patterns of

muscle groups, their support of each other, their particular roles, and
the necessity for changes in roles have not been addressed in detail.

In the human dietary requirements have been studied in depth.
Each study 'discovers' a 'new' quirk: fats are in, fats are out; load
carbohydrate precompetition on Day 1, do not on Day 2, do not on
Day 3, and so on. All this probably means that metabolism varies in
each individual, as does movement. Despite the extensive research on
humans there are no definitive 'rules', only guidelines.

Muscle action operates the bone leverage system and movement
results. Each equine sport activity demands differing movement
patterns, thus the workload demand upon muscle groups varies with
each sport. The human only has two legs and two paces; the horse has
four legs and six paces – walk, trot, canter, gallop, triple and pace. It is
hardly surprising that the site of a muscle injury is difficult to detect in
the equine. In the human the analysis of muscle activity during the
movements demanded by various sports is very comprehensive, thus
enabling the masseur to detect injury sites more easily. Also many

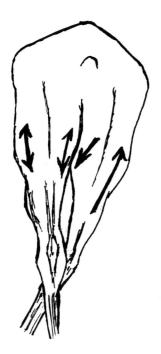
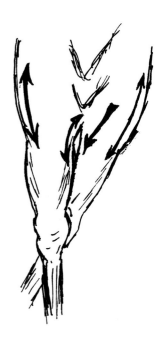

Fig. 8.2 The lateral work demanded in dressage requires the groups of muscles, the
abductors and adductors to work in an active role, even though their normal role is of
support.

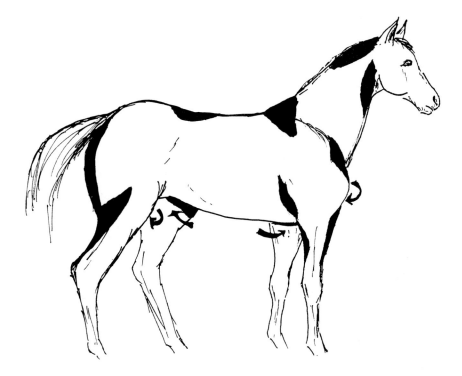

Fig. 8.3 Dressage stress areas.

injuries are common to a particular sport. The same principles apply to equine competitive sport. Each discipline creates its own particular movement sequences and widely differing demands upon the musculo-skeletal system. These differ not only sport from sport, but also from the demands of general riding for pleasure.

Areas of stress which *may* require attention are suggested for each of the common disciplines in an endeavour to assist those wishing to help their horses.

These are suggestions only; they are based upon the author's experience. Common sense and close observation will indicate any changes required.

Dressage

Dressage even at Novice level is a very demanding sport, a factor often overlooked, particularly as many dressage horses derive from the various breeds of warm bloods, and are large and apparently strong.

The visual impression is often misleading as the animals are slow to mature, both physically and mentally.

The work demands precise elastic movements (see Fig. 8.2), many of which are vertical. These are combined with lateral movements, unnatural sudden changes of tempo and of stride length, and the necessity to 'hold' an outline throughout, be it for a schooling session or a test.

Areas of stress (see Fig. 8.3)

- The neck, the area just behind the poll in particular.
- The back, the area just forward of the loins beneath the rider's seat in particular.
- The shoulder and forearm muscles.
- The muscles of the second thigh (gaskin).
- The hind limb flexors (retractors).
- The adductors and abductors of front and hind limbs.

Stretches

- All stretches.

Driving

The horse must pull, rather than carry, a load. Over uneven terrain this necessitates the ability to 'lean' into the harness after planting the lead leg.

The muscular efforts may be influenced by the way the horse works with others. For example, when driven to a four-in-hand the wheelers (the horses nearest the vehicle) have to sit into the breaching to assist the brake as the vehicle rolls downhill, whereas the leaders are responsible for the initiation of an uphill drag. If an animal's partner is lazy or slow to react one horse may lean inward trying to do the work of two. This will place uneven demands upon the limbs and body mass creating uneven muscle fatigue.

Areas of stress (see Fig. 8.4)

- The shoulders.
- The muscles of the forearms.
- The quarters.
- The muscles of the second thigh (gaskin).

- The mid back.
- The poll, mid neck, and withers if a bearing rein is used.

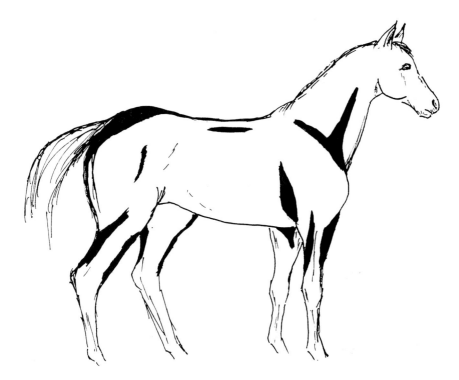

Fig. 8.4 Driving stress areas.

Stretches

- All leg stretches.

Endurance, long distance

The sport requires the horse to achieve an ability to maintain a moderate pace, across a varied terrain, over long distances while carrying a rider. In competition the level of fatigue is influenced by atmospheric temperature and humidity. If both are high some level of dehydration will result and the muscle tissues will be in an *abnormal state*.

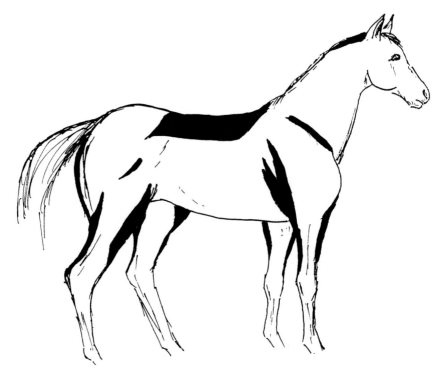

Fig. 8.5 Endurance, long distance stress areas.

Areas of stress (see Fig. 8.5)

- The back from withers to loins.
- The limb muscles.
- Areas within the shoulders and quarters, varying depending upon the terrain and footing.

Stretches

- All back stretches.
- Limb stretches appropriate to the area if stiffness or pain is discovered.

Flat racing

The horse is required to attain maximum speed from a stand still, to settle to and maintain that pace over the distance judged the most suitable by the trainer, and then to draw on energy reserves to achieve maximum plus speed at the end of the race.

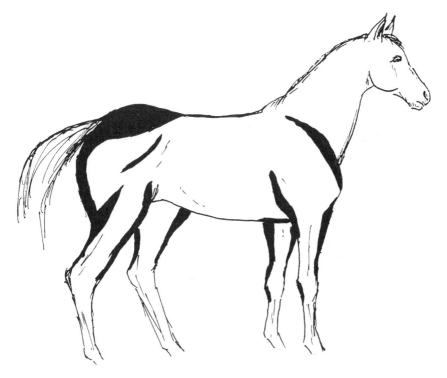

Fig. 8.6 Flat racing stress areas.

Areas of stress (see Fig. 8.6)

- The forelimb muscles.
- The back of the shoulders.
- The loins.
- The quarters, flanks and hindlimb muscles.

Stretches

- Forelimb stretches.
- Neck stretches.
- Back stretches.

Hurdling

The horse is required to travel fast, accelerating from walk to gallop and to negotiate a series of obstacles, all of a consistent width and height. These may be sited on the flat or on a slope. The animal will meet the ground with an outstretched forelimb.

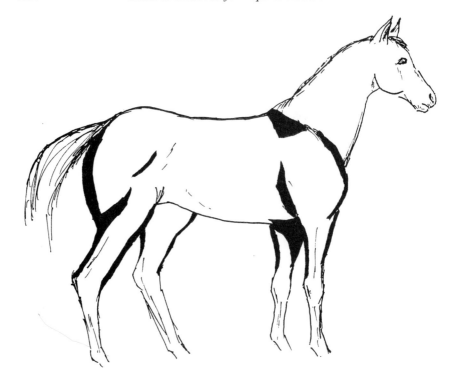

Fig. 8.7 Hurdling: stress areas.

Areas of stress (see Fig. 8.7)

- The forelimbs.
- The shoulders.
- The quarters.
- The loins.

Stretches

- Forelimb stretches.

National hunt, timber racing, point-to-point racing, team chasing
The horse is required to accelerate from a walk to a moderate gallop
negotiating a series of fences, of varying heights and widths, sited on
the flat, on a slope, on a corner, and to maintain a good pace both up
and down hill, round bends and elbows over distances from $1^1/_2$ miles
upward. Falls are common.

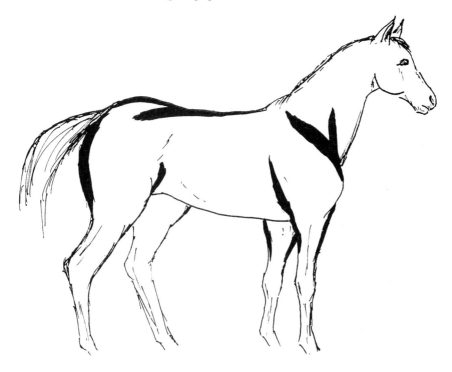

Fig. 8.8 National hunt stress areas.

Areas of stress (see Fig.8.8)

- Shoulders.
- Quarters.
- Loins.

Stretches

- All head and neck stretches.
- All back stretches.
- Shoulder and knee stretches.

Polo, barrel racing, cutting, roping
All these disciplines require the horse to be agile; they all require the animal to 'spin' on one hock, sitting on the pivot hock and then to transfer its weight in a manner which allows it to race forward at speed. Rider balance is another factor to be considered when searching for stress areas.

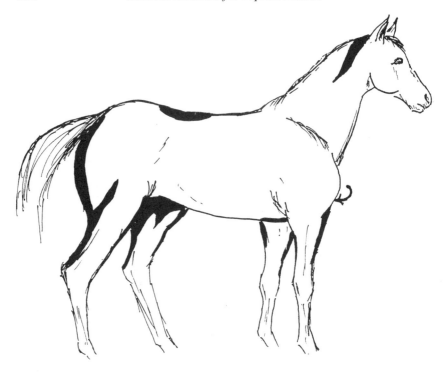

Fig. 8.9 Polo stress areas.

Areas of stress (see Fig. 8.9)

- Head and neck.
- Hindquarters
- Hamstrings
- Hock muscles.
- The abductors and adductors.

Stretches

- All stretches.

Show jumping

The horse is required to negotiate a number of obstacles, many of which are combinations, at a moderate pace. Often the jumps will be taken on a turn and courses necessitate frequent changes of leg. The horse needs athletic ability, speed, muscle power and a consistent precision in its movement sequences. Sudden bursts of power to achieve elevation are required.

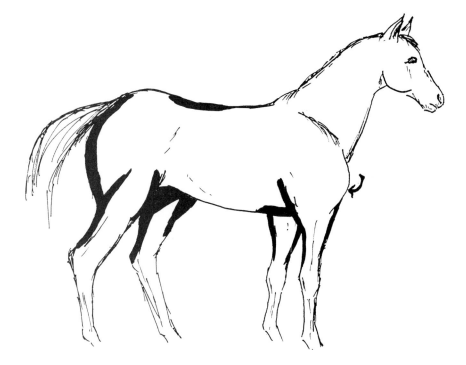

Fig. 8.10 Showjumping stress areas.

Areas of stress (see Fig. 8.10)

- The hindlimbs.
- The quarters.
- The loins.
- The abductors and adductors.

Stretches

- All stretches.

Trotting or harness racing

The horse pulls a light racing cart carrying the driver. The gait maybe at trot or the animal may be so harnessed that it paces, with the head positioned high and held with a rein.

Areas of stress (see Fig. 8.5)

- The head and neck.
- The hindlimbs.
- The mid back.

Stretches

- Head and neck stretches.
- All back stretches.

Eventing

Dressage, cross-country skills and showjumping are all combined in an equine triathlon. The phases may all take place during one day or be spread over three days. The sport tests obedience, stamina and versatility.

Areas of stress (see Figs. 8.3, 8.8 and 8.10)

- These will depend upon individual conformation; each horse must be assessed separately.

Stretches

- All stretches.

While massage and stretching are of value whenever they are used, their greatest value is both prior to and during competitions, provided the horse has been introduced to all the massage techniques and stretch routines over a period of time.

It is the height of stupidity to vary a routine at the last minute. Ten days is the minimum period in which to familiarize the horse with a set of new experiences.

Pleasurable relaxation should be the end result, so if a horse resents either massage and/or passive stretches reassess the animal.

9 Passive Stretches

Introduction

No human athletic training programme is complete without the inclusion of a regime of stretching exercises. Stretching achieves suppleness of all the structures surrounding the joints and within the muscles moving the joints. The stretching of joints and their supporting structures will ensure the full range of available movement is achieved and maintained. It must be remembered that joints are designed and fashioned in a manner which allows for a pre-ordained range of movement. Trying to exceed this range, by employing force, is *not* the idea behind passive stretching.

The aim of stretching is to enhance athletic ability. Muscles can be likened to finely tempered springs. If springs are kept well oiled they achieve maximum work with minimum effort. However, if they are allowed to get rusty and lose their recoil, the story is very different. Stretched muscles respond like oiled springs.

The horse cannot be taught stretches and then expected to perform them by himself. Horses may stretch when they get up after lying down. They usually tuck the nose toward the chest and stretch one or other hind leg backward. Some stretch both front legs forward after being girthed up, but regular stretching needs to be performed by the masseur. The owner or groom can be taught the correct procedure if appropriate.

General points

(1) Tissues are less likely to tear or be damaged by overstretching if they are warm, so stretch *after massage*.
(2) Study the anatomy of the joints before stretching.

(3)   Hold the limb in a manner comfortable for both you and the horse.

(4)   Position yourself so that you can move the limb without straining your back.

(5)   Never use sudden forceful thrusts.

(6)   Stretch slowly to the full extent of available range. At the first hint of resistance stop, massage the resistant structures and try it again.

(7)   Stretch using a gentle traction. This will ensure that the elongation achieved will, in part, remain. Bouncy stretching (pull, release; pull, release), while increasing elasticity at the time, can cause a later loss of elasticity, rather than an increase.

(8)   Repeat each movement five times.

(9)   Desist if the animal shows obvious resentment, or if the muscles appear to 'guard' by tensing.

(10)   At the end of *each* stretch allow the limb to reposition normally.

Head and neck

Full passive movement by the operator of a horse's neck are impossible to achieve because of the weight and resistance created by the tonic neck reflexes.

Neck suppling is achieved with the aid of a carrot, polo mint or other gastronomic inducement.

Top neck stretch (see Plate 9.1)
Have the horse standing square, wearing a head collar but not restrained, offer him the chosen bribe, slowly move it down his chest and then between his front legs. As his head follows your hand so he will stretch the neck structures from poll to withers.

Side neck stretching (see Plate 9.2)
Have the horse stand square, offer the bribe and slowly move it back toward his ribs. Repeat on the opposite side. A horse should be able to reach halfway down the rib cage with ease.

Check to ensure the neck bends evenly throughout. A badly tilted head or inability to get muzzle to ribs needs investigation.

Check for muscle tension from poll to withers on both sides of the neck. Massage any hypertensive painful areas before further attempts.

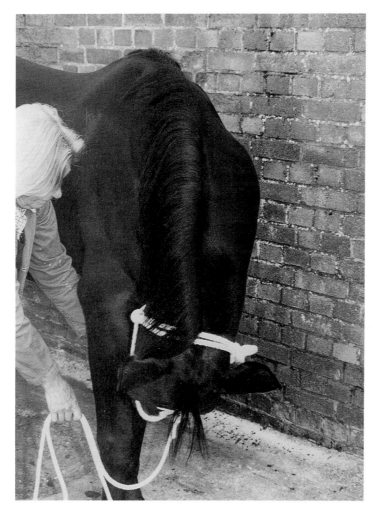

Plate 9.1 Top neck stretch.

The shoulder

It is impossible to stretch the shoulder joint as an independent structure. The joint is part of a unit consisting of the (scapula) shoulderblade and the elbow joint – the site of articulation between the humerus and the uppermost bones of the forelimb (the fused radius and ulna) (see Fig. 5.2).

The movements described anatomically are protraction (forward or extension) and retraction (bending or flexion). Both of these involve

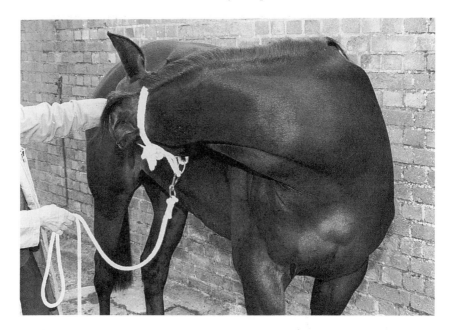

Plate 9.2 Side neck stretch.

the elbow joint. Articulation between the hemispherical head of the humerus and the shallow acetabulum of the scapula comprises a ball and socket joint, so theoretically rotation is possible. As the horse does not require such a complex movement, the muscle groups on the inner and outer aspects of the joint (the abductors and adductors) act mainly as stabilizers for the shoulder complex in the natural state. The lateral movements demanded in dressage require unusual activity in these two sets of muscles.

Protraction stretch I (knee at 90° angle) (see Plate 9.3)

- Stand beside the horse, slightly in front of the shoulder, pick up the foreleg in the normal manner as if you were about to pick out the foot.
- Transfer the hands and grasp the forearm allowing the knee joint to bend and hang loose.
- Move the limb forward through its available range and then back to the normal position.
- As the horse relaxes add increased traction at the end of each excursion of the limb.

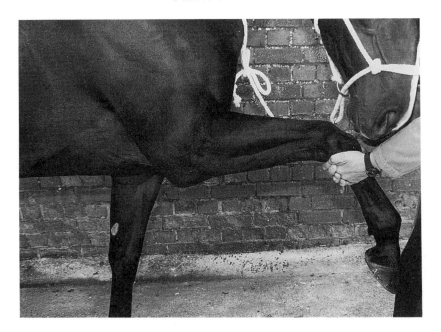

Plate 9.3 Protraction stretch I.

Protraction stretch II (knee extended) (see Plate 9.4)

● Stand well in front of the horse and slightly to one side.
● Grasp the forelimb behind the fetlock joint and stretch the whole limb forward and upward to the end of range.
● As the horse relaxes, gently increase the force applied at the end of the movement.

This stretch can be achieved by using a wide woollen leg bandage (wrap). The unrolled bandage is placed so that its centre is behind the fetlock and the masseur holds the two ends pulling the limb forward by the traction achieved when the bandage ends are pulled away from the horse (see Plate 9.4). N.B.: This also stretches the knee in extension.

Retraction stretch I (knee flexed (see Plate 9.5)

● Stand beside the horse level with the shoulder. Pick up the forelimb in the normal manner as if you were about to pick out the foot.
● Grasp the cannon bone and flex the knee.

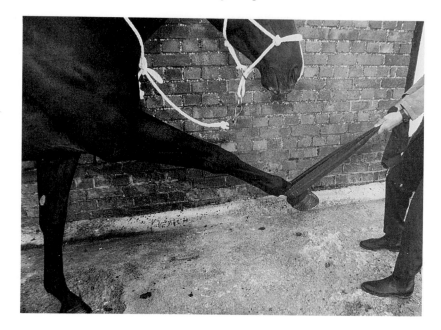

Plate 9.4 Protraction stretch II.

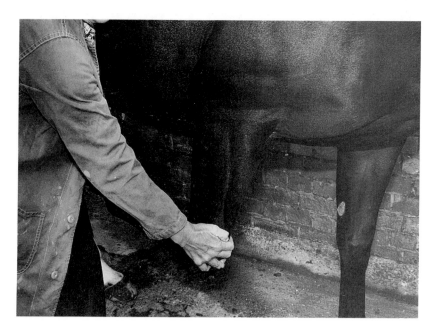

Plate 9.5 Retraction stretch I.

- Place one hand over the knee and push the limb complex backwards to the end of the available range.
- As the horse relaxes increase the pressure when at the limit of backward movement.

Retraction stretch II (knee extended) (see Plate 9.6)

- Stand well behind the horse's shoulder.
- Grasp the forelimb around the fetlock joint.
- Stretch the entire limb backward and slightly upward.
- As the horse relaxes increase the pressure at the limit of movement both up and backward.

Adduction stretch (knee extended) (see Plate 9.7)
Actually Stretches adductors, but limb is abducted
- Stand and position the limb as for Protraction stretch II.
- At full forward stretch pull the limb outward away from the animal's body.

Do not force – stretch *carefully*.

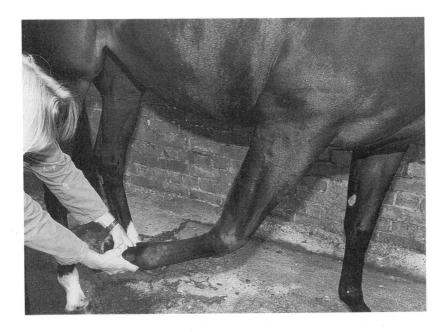

Plate 9.6 Retraction stretch II.

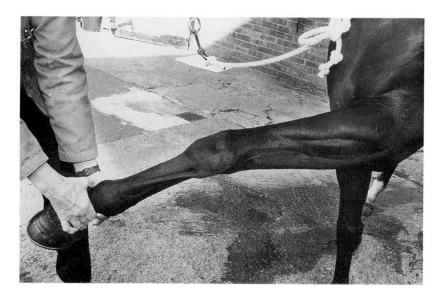

Plate 9.7 Adduction stretch.

Abduction stretch (knee extended)

● Stand and position the limb as for Protraction stretch II.
● At full forward stretch pull the limb across the front of the body.

Do not force – stretch *carefully*.

The knee

The knee of the horse is a hinge joint. Its muscles and construction allow for flexion (bending) and extension (straightening) and small bones which comprise the joint glide within the joint during movement. Head-on slow motion films taken with the horse galloping demonstrate the entire limb rotating in mid-air flight as the forelimb stretches forward with the foot feeling for the ground.

The knee joint cannot be manually stretched to full extension. Protraction stretch II achieves extension but is approximately 15° off full extension.

Knee flexion I (see Plate 9.8)

● Stand beside the horse and grasp the cannon bone.

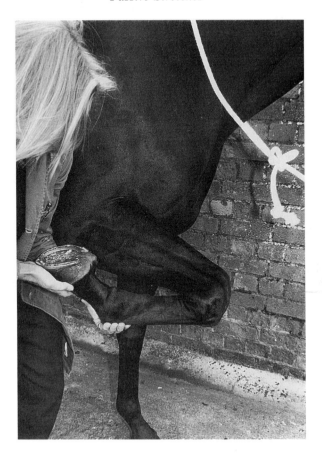

Plate 9.8 Knee flexion I.

- Bend the knee until the back of the fetlock touches the underside of the forearm.
- The forearm must be parallel to the ground.
- Move the cannon bone inward until the back of the fetlock is no longer in contact.
- Push the cannon gently upward.
- Repeat but pull the cannon outward.

Ten to fifteen degrees of extra movement will be achieved.

N.B. Some horses have restriction of these movements following knee surgery, or if arthritic changes have occurred. In these cases stretch *very carefully*.

Knee stretch II

- Proceed as for Knee flexion I.
- Stop flexion approximately 15° before the back of the fetlock touches the underside of the forearm.
- Push the cannon toward the centre of the body, then pull outward away from the centre of the body.

Never force knee movements.

Fetlocks

The extension excursion achieved within the fetlock joints of both the front and hind limbs when either limit is fully protracted and the entire body weight of the animal is supported on the limb cannot be achieved manually.

Fetlock stretch

- Stand the grasp the limb exactly as when picking out the foot.
- Hold the foot in one hand and the cannon above the joint in the other.
- Move the foot up and down with overpressure at the end of each movement.

N.B.: This stretch is particularly useful following fracture of a sesamoid.

The hip joint

The hip is a powerful ball and socket joint (see Fig. 5.3), as is the shoulder joint, but the hip joint exhibits a construction design of considerably greater strength, with a deep bowl-type socket (acetabulum) containing the massive half spherical femoral head. The head is attached by an internal as well as external ligaments. The movements at the joint are primarily flexion and extension, body mass, muscle and ligament placement limiting range to ensure safety and strength.

The hip, stifle and hock joints must be considered as a whole. Individual stretches are not possible and even if they were the complexity of the unit and its function during motion demand synchronized movement patterns dependent on the balance of one to the other bone levers, as well as the associated muscle power and excursion. Safety and limitation of movement are partially achieved by ligament length. While the hip is an independent joint within the complex, hock and stifle movement are coupled together. Flexion or extension in either one of the two immediately causes the same movement to occur in its partner. This feature is ensured by virtue of tendinous bands within local structures, in particular, peroneus tertius. The movements within the complex are also very dependent upon the stability of the stifle joint. Problems such as 'stifle locking', or orthopaedic disease such as cystic conditions, transmit extra strain upon the hock joint, the hardest working joint in the horse.

Hindlimb stretch I (see Plate 9.9)

- Stand level with the midline of the horse facing toward the tail.
- Grasp the limb at mid cannon and pull the limb forward and up.
- When the horse settles increase the traction force.

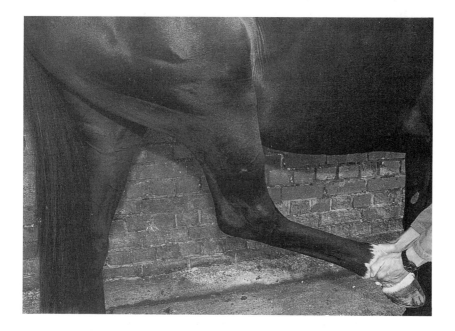

Plate 9.9 Hindlimb stretch I.

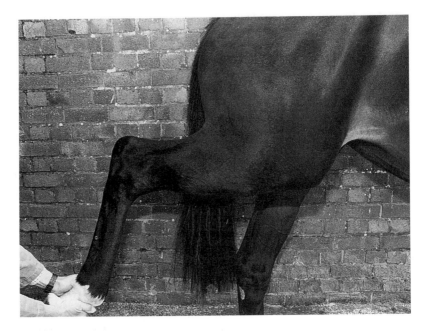

Plate 9.10 Hindlimb stretch II.

Hindlimb stretch II (see Plate 9.10)
Do not attempt this stretch on any horse known to kick.

- Stand behind the horse, slightly to one side facing the quarters.
- Grasp the cannon bone and pull the limb complex backward.
- If the horse settles increase traction at the end of movement range.

The range of movement in the joints of the hindlimb is less than those of the front limb. Neither hip, stifle or hock can extend to a 90° angle, and flexion is limited by construction and body mass.

The back

The horse's back is considered, by horsemen, to stretch from withers to loins. Remarkably little attention is paid either to the anatomical features or to the biomechanics. This may, in part, be due to the widely differing opinions of the experts. There is just as much confusion regarding the human back! However, there are certain known features and in order to understand the back the movements must be discussed. Anatomically they consist of:

- Rounding the back, dorsiflexion
- Hollowing the back, ventroflexion
- Side bending, side flexion

Certain movements demand axial rotations. The construction allows for this, for if it totally blocked rotation, the components would break (fracture) under the strain.

The horse *does not* perform any back movements as a voluntary action. He will bend his neck sideways to bite his sides if troubled by an irritation, and if the irritation is on his flank he stretches his hindlimb forward toward his bent neck. Pain in the back does not cause the horse, as it does the human, to rub the area or stretch by hollowing, straightening or arching. The horse may attempt to influence the pain by rolling or kicking back.

The horse does not stand in a field or box deliberating exercising as a daily activity, with its back rounding, hollowing or bending sideways. However, if the correct reflex areas are stimulated the movements occur as a *reflex*, rather than a *voluntary* action.

Consider the horse's back as a sprung girder, with minor collapse and recoil available to absorb the concussion generated during movement as the limbs meet the ground. Anatomically the back begins not at the withers, but between the shoulder blades at the site of the first thoracic vertebrae (see Fig. 9.1). A main part of the suspension system lies between the front legs where the forward ribs attach to the breastbone (sternum). Problems within this complex will affect the entire back for the greatest amount of dorso-ventral movement occurs in two areas: at the first thoracic vertebral complex just described and at the junction of the loins to quarters, the lumbo-sacral junction (Townsend, Leach & Fritz, University of Saskatchewan).

Recent work in Japan (private communication) using implanted electrodes to monitor the muscle activity of the back during walk, trot, canter and gallop over ground with and without a rider demonstrates differences both in movement range and in the muscle firing patterns. The added rider weight causes some muscle groups to adopt a partially static, rather than a fully active role. The work, still in early stages, suggests the ability of the back to work when ridden in a manner which mimics that of the riderless horse, requires great attention to

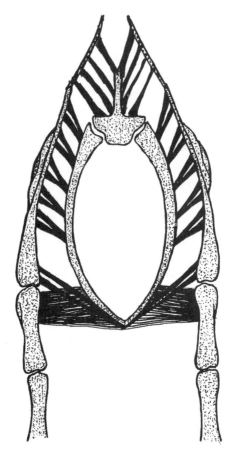

Fig. 9.1 The first thoracic vertebrae and the first pair of ribs suspended between the pair of shoulder blades (scapulae).

saddle fit. This is not a new concept. Smith in 1882 wrote a treatise on saddle fit and designed the cavalry saddle which is still in use over 100 years later. Rider weight needs to be distributed over as large an area as is practical via flat panels that mould to the contours of the equine back. The gutter between the panels bridging the centre of the back should be wide allowing for recoil and thus shock absorption within the bone complex of the spine.

Back stretches cannot be performed passively by the masseur, but movements to supple the back can be achieved by stimulating reflex points. The horse must be relaxed, preferably following a massage session, for all the suppling responses.

Rounding (dorsiflexion)

- Stand with one hand on the withers and place the other hand on the centre line just behind the girth and just forward of the umbilicus.
- Press firmly upward. The horse will raise his back and lower the head.

Hollowing (ventroflexion)

- Stand by the side of the horse.
- Run the hands along the back, one on either side of the centre about one hand's span from the centre.
- Position the hands forward of the loins, approximately where the rider's seat bones would meet the saddle if it were in place.
- Press firmly down.
- The horse will hollow the back and raise the head.

Side flexion

- Run the tips of the fingers along one side of the back from withers to loins a half hand span from the centre of the back.
- Press firmly as the fingers move back toward the quarters.
- The horse will bend away from the pressure.
- Repeat on the opposite side of the back.

Desist if the horse shows any resentment to pressure or the muscle goes into spasm to 'guard' an area. This reaction indicates there is a problem which needs to be addressed.

It is interesting to note that the head raise/back hollowing reflex can be activated by the pressure caused by a rider sitting too deep. The horse is forced to dip the back and raise the head by a reflex over which is has no control – its brain makes this occur as an automatic response. When this happens the position of back and neck is then incorrect and outline is lost.

All too often instead of addressing saddle fit and rider weight distribution, a restraint designed to lower the head by pressure on the sensitive bars of the mouth and/or on the sensitive poll is used to force the head down. Small wonder the animal becomes confused: its brain is giving one command, and the creature's pain another with tension as the immediate result. When this occurs the animal cannot work in a relaxed supple manner.

To achieve flexibility by passive stretching requires time and patience. Conformation must be considered along with muscle build. Do not expect exactly similar responses from each animal – after all not all humans can touch their toes with ease!

Do not 'overdo' the routine. The concept that 'the more the exercises are done the better' is false. Enough is enough, too much is bad. It is better to do too little than too much. It will take approximately three weeks before any improvement in tight structures is observed. Once this is achieved a weekly maintenance stretch will be sufficient to retain flexibility.

To recap, muscles are similar to groups of beautifully tempered balanced springs. Your horse depends upon healthy muscles for effective movements and healthy muscles require a strong bone structure both to act as a leverage system and as an anchor for muscle attachment. Other essentials are systems for a command, delivery of food, removal of waste, repair facilities, and temperature control.

You can aid your horse by ensuring that it has access to a dietary intake as palatable, natural and well balanced as is possible to ensure both general and muscle health. By massage and passive stretching you can help muscles, which in a natural state are continually active, to remain pliable and therefore efficient in the unnatural lifestyle most horses have been forced, through domestication, to adopt. Evolutionary changes do not occur rapidly – horses still need space to run free if they so wish.

General Bibliography

Clayton, H.M. (1991) *Conditioning Sport Horses*. Sport Horse Publications, Saskatchewan.

Cook, W.R. (1989) *Speed in the Racehorse*. Russell Maerdink Co Ltd, USA.

Denoix, J.M. (1992) *Biomécanique et Travail Physique du Cheval*. RCS Versailles, Paris.

Denoix, J.M. & Pailloux, J.P. (1989) *Kinesithérapie du Cheval*. Maloine, Paris.

Giniaux, D. (1993) *Soulagez Votre Cheval aux Doigts*. Favre, Paris.

Johnson, A.M. (1994) *Equine Medical Disorders*, 2nd edn. Blackwell Scientific Publications, Oxford.

Jones, W.E. (1989) *Equine Sports Medicine*. Lea and Febiger, USA.

Snow, D.H. & Vogel, C.J. (1987) *Equine Fitness*. David and Charles, Newton Abbot, Devon.

Glossary

Abdomen: that portion of the body which lies between the chest and the pelvis.

Abduction: a drawing away from the median plane of the body.

Absorption: the uptake of substances into or across tissues.

Acupuncture: a Chinese science of influencing the body systems.

Adduction: a drawing towards the median plane of the body.

Aerobic: functions which can only occur in the presence of an oxygen molecule.

Amino acid: the body proteins necessary for all functions are composed of amino acids; some are manufactured by the body, others are extracted from food.

Anaerobic: function which occurs in the absence of oxygen.

Anion: an ion that conducts negatively charged electricity.

Anterior: situated in front of, or in the forward part of, an organ; towards the head end of the body.

Arteriole: a very small branch of the arterial system connecting to a capillary.

Artery: a blood vessel containing arterial blood charged with cells, oxygen and fuel. Arteries are sited to allow the passage of blood away from the heart.

Atrophy: wasting away of a normally developed organ or tissue due to degeneration of cells.

Avascular: not supplied with blood vessels.

Avulsion: the tearing away of part of a structure.

Balance: (Chinese concept) the necessity for harmony within all systems of living organisms.

Bifurcation: the site where a single structure divides into two branches.

Bilateral: prefix 'bi' relates to two, thus bilateral denotes both lateral sides.

Blood pressure: the pressure of blood on the walls of the arteries, dependent on the energy of the heart action, the elasticity of the walls of the arteries, and the volume and viscosity of the blood.

Bone: a dense connective tissue that forms the skeleton.

Bone marrow: the internal cavities of the bones act as factories manufacturing cells.

Bronchus, bronchi: either or both of the two main branches of the trachea, one going to each lung.

Bursa: a sac or sac-like cavity filled with fluid and situated at places in the tissues at which friction would otherwise develop.

Bursitis: an inflammation of the bursa, occasionally accompanied by the formation of a calcific deposit in the underlying tendon.

Capillary: a minute vessel, with walls only one cell thick enabling the exchange of all components within the body's structures; the blood in the network is delivered by the arterioles and removed by the venules.

Capsule: the tissue surrounding a joint and assisting in joint lubrication.

Cardiac: pertaining to the heart.

Cardiac cycle: the actions of the heart during one complete heart beat.

Cartilage: a dense connective tissue found at the working end of the bones; also found in the intravertebral disc of the ear, the larynx, the trachea and the walls of the larger bronchi.

Catalyst: a substance capable of changing a chemical reaction and yet itself remaining unchanged.

Cation: an ion that conducts positively charged electricity.

Caudel: the area behind the central area of the horse's body.

Cell: all living organisms are composed of cells, each cell type is specialized to perform a particular function. Cells are the basic units of all life.

Chelate: the process by which the body renders minerals usable.

Ch'i: Chinese term for energy.

Chronic: long-term, continued; not acute.

Chronos: comparative history arranged in a chronological manner.

Conformation: the shape or contour of the body or body structures.

Congenital: existing at and usually before birth; referring to conditions that may or may not be inherited.

Connective tissue: the tissue which binds together other tissues into functional units. Variations in the composition of the basic elements give rise to a variety of functional differences.

Contusion: a bruise or injury incurred without breaking the skin.

Cranium: the bones enclosing and protecting the brain. *adj. cranial.*

Diagnosis: identifying a disease from its characteristics and/or causative agent; distinguishing one disease from another.

Diaphragm: the muscular membrane separating the abdominal and chest cavities.

Dilatation: the condition of being dilated or stretched beyond normal dimensions.

Dilation: a stretching or expansion.

Dislocation: the displacement of any part, usually referring to a bone.

Distal: a point further from the centre of the body.

Distension: the state of being swollen or enlarged from internal pressure.

Dorsal: pertaining to the back or denoting a position more towards the back surface than some other point of reference.

Dynamization: a process in the preparation of homoeopathic remedies.

Dysfunction: disturbance or impairing of the function of an organ.

Electrolyte: a substance composed of ions, electrolytes regulate the conduction of the electrical charges within the body. They are lost by excessive sweating and diarrhoea. When severely diminished electrolytes need to be replaced by giving the appropriate substance by mouth or intravenous drip.

Enzyme: the catalyst of a biochemical reaction.

Epidermis: the outermost layer of skin which is not supplied with blood vessels.

Epithelium: the covering of internal and external surfaces of the body, including the lining of vessels and other small cavities; it consists of cells joined together by small amounts of cementing substances.

Excretion: the removal of metabolic waste from the body.

Extension: a movement that brings a limb into a straight line.

Extensor: any muscle that extends a joint.

Extra cellular: outside the confines of the cells.

Fen: a Chinese measurement: 10 *fen* = 1 *tsun.*

Fibrosis: the formation of fibrous tissue.

Flexion: the act of bending.

Fossa: a hollow or depressed area.

Haematoma: an accumulation of blood within the tissues that clots to form a solid swelling.

Haemoglobin: the oxygen-carrying protein pigment of the red blood cells.

Haemorrhage: the escape of blood from the vessels; bleeding.

Hyperextend: extreme or excessive extension of a limb.

Hyperflexion: forcible overflexion of a limb or part.

Hypersensitivity: a state of altered activity in which the body reacts with an exaggerated response to a foreign agent.

Insertion: the point of attachment of a muscle (e.g. to a bone).

Inspiration: the act of inhaling or drawing air into the lungs.

Intracellular: interactions taking place with a cell.

Intravenous: within a vein.

Involuntary: performed independently of the will, contravolitional; as in an involuntary muscle.

Ischaemia: inadequate circulatory flow caused by constriction of the local blood vessels.

Joint: an articulation; the place of union or junction between two or more bones of the skeleton.

Larynx: the structure of muscle and cartilage located at the top of the trachea and below the root of the tongue; the 'voice box'.

Lateral: pertaining to a side or outer surface; a position further from the midline of the body or of a structure.

Ligament: a band of fibrous tissue that connects bones or cartilages.

Lumbar: pertaining to the loins, the part of the back between the thorax and pelvis.

Lymph: a transparent yellowish liquid containing mostly white blood cells and derived from tissue fluids.

Medial: pertaining to the middle or inner surface; a position closer to the midline of the body or of a structure.

Meridians: conceptual paths within the body considered by the Chinese to interlink all body organs.

Mobility: the ability to move.

Mother tincture: a term used to denote the source of a remedy in the Back Flower remedies.

Muscle: an organ which by contraction produced the movements of an animal organism.

Muscle tremor: an involuntary trembling or quivering of a muscle.

Necrosis: death of a cell or group of cells which is in contact with living tissue.

Nerves: cord-like structures, visible to the naked eye, comprising a collection of nerve fibres which convey impulses between a part of the central nervous system and some other region of the body.

Non-vascular: not supplied with blood vessels.

Nosode: material extracted from the product of a condition or disease and used to effect a cure.

Oedema: excessive accumulation of fluid in the body tissues.

Optic: pertaining to the eye.

Ossify: to change or develop into bone.

Palpation: the act of feeling with the hand.

Plasma: the liquid portion of the blood, containing the suspended particulate components.

Platelets: disc-shaped structures found in the blood of all mammals and chiefly known for their role in the blood coagulation: also called *blood platelets.* (See also *Thrombocytes.*)

Plexus: a network of lymphatic vessels, nerves, veins or arteries.

Point: the term used to describe the area where acupressure or acupuncture should be administered.

Posterior: situated behind, or in the back of, a structure; towards the rear end of the body.

Potency: required dilution of a homoeopathic remedy.

Prognosis: the prospect of recovery from a disease or injury.

Progressive: advancing, going from bad to worse; advancing in severity.

Proud flesh: excessive granulation tissue.

Pulmonary: pertaining to the lungs.

Pulse: rhythmic throbbing of an artery which may be felt with the finger; caused by blood forced through the vessel by contractions of the heart.

Red blood cells: haemoglobin-carrying corpuscles in the blood, that transport oxygen.

Regeneration: the natural renewal of a structure, as of a tissue part.

Remedy: the term used in homoeopathy to describe the appropriate restorative for a diagnosed problem.

Rotation: the process of turning around an axis.

Scar tissue: tissue remaining after the healing of a wound or other morbid process.

Septum: a dividing wall or partition.

Subacute: somewhat acute, between acute and chronic.

Subluxation: an incomplete or partial dislocation.

Succussion: a process of shaking, essential in the preparation of homoeopathic remedies.

Supraspinous: above a spine or spinous process.

Thrombocytes: blood platelets.

Tsun: a Chinese term for measurement (see also *Fen*).

Vein: a vessel through which the blood passes from various organs or parts back to the heart.

Venous: pertaining to the veins.

Virus: a particle that uses cells as a host and replicates within chosen cells; the effects of the replication are toxic and cause side effects toxic to the main host. Vaccines do control some viral invasions, antibiotics are ineffective but may be needed to control secondary infections.

Voluntary: accompanied in accordance with the will.

Yang: Chinese term for positive energy.

Yin: Chinese term for negative energy.

Index